Social Work Practice and End-of-Life Care

T0200595

This book draws together the learning of a wide range of social workers and other professionals engaged in end-of-life care who recognise that dying is essentially a social experience and want to tailor a personal, professional and societal response accordingly. Through a systemic lens, the book explores the nature and experience of living and dying in the United Kingdom today and considers the ways in which social workers and others may want to work with people who are affected by a diagnosis of a life-threatening condition.

The contributors offer rich and contemporary perspectives on death, dying and loss, reflective of their different approaches and interests. The insights of the book are timely, given the growing levels and changing nature of needs for people who are coming to the end of their life in the United Kingdom and beyond, and the related requirements for compassionate, personalised and holistic care within the increasingly professionalised arena of health and social care.

This book will be of interest to social work practitioners, students and others committed to psychosocial support of people who are dying or bereaved, and who want to consider how to provide this support most effectively. Professionals who are interested in working alongside social workers to deliver high-quality end-of-life care will also find this publication useful.

The chapters in this book were originally published as a special issue of the *Journal of Social Work Practice*.

Heather Richardson is Joint Chief Executive of St Christopher's Hospice, London, and Honorary Professor in Palliative Care at Lancaster University, UK. She is a nurse, and has held clinical, managerial and leadership roles in hospice/palliative care over the last thirty years. Her PhD focused on people's experience of day hospice.

Gillian Chowns is a social worker by profession, and has practised, lectured and researched in palliative care. Her PhD examined the experience of children living with the life-threatening illness of a parent. She is Chair of the Board of Trustees of Palliative Care Works, a charity offering education, training and mentoring in resource-poor settings.

Social Work Practice and
End-of-Life Care

Edited by
Heather Richardson and Gillian Chowns

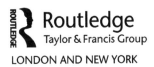
Routledge
Taylor & Francis Group

LONDON AND NEW YORK

First published 2018 by Routledge

2 Park Square, Milton Park, Abingdon, Oxfordshire OX14 4RN
52 Vanderbilt Avenue, New York, NY 10017

Routledge is an imprint of the Taylor & Francis Group, an informa business

First issued in paperback 2020

Introduction - Chapter 6 & Chapter 8 © 2018 GAPS
Chapter 7 © 2018 Jason Davidson

British Library Cataloguing in Publication Data
A catalogue record for this book is available from the British Library

ISBN 13: 978-0-8153-8312-3 (hbk)
ISBN 13: 978-0-367-59290-5 (pbk)

Typeset in Perpetua
by diacriTech, Chennai

Publisher's Note
The publisher accepts responsibility for any inconsistencies that may have arisen during the
conversion of this book from journal articles to book chapters, namely the possible inclusion
of journal terminology.

Disclaimer
Every effort has been made to contact copyright holders for their permission to reprint
material in this book. The publishers would be grateful to hear from any copyright holder
who is not here acknowledged and will undertake to rectify any errors or omissions in future
editions of this book.

Contents

CONTENTS

Citation Information

The chapters in this book were originally published in the *Journal of Social Work Practice*, volume 30, issue 2 (June 2016). When citing this material, please use the original page numbering for each article, as follows:

Chapter 6
Working with Communities to Develop Resilience in End of Life and Bereavement Care: Hospices, Schools and Health Promoting Palliative Care
Sally Paul
Journal of Social Work Practice, volume 30, issue 2 (June 2016) pp. 187–201

Chapter 7
Does the Culture of Modern Day Palliative Care Social Work Leave Room for Leadership?
Jason Davidson
Journal of Social Work Practice, volume 30, issue 2 (June 2016) pp. 203–218

Chapter 8
Schwartz Rounds® – Promoting Compassionate Care and Healthy Organisations
Anne Cullen
Journal of Social Work Practice, volume 30, issue 2 (June 2016) pp. 219–228

For any permission-related enquiries please visit:
http://www.tandfonline.com/page/help/permissions

Notes on Contributors

Lesley Adshead is a visiting lecturer at St Christopher's Hospice, UK. Her research interests include social care at end of life and social work education. Her publications include *Palliative Care, Social Work and Service Users: Making Life Possible* (2007).

Rebecca Chaddock is Head of Supportive Care at St Columba's Hospice in Edinburgh, Scotland. She has been Vice Chair of the Association of Palliative Care Social Workers since 2010, and is co-author of *The Role of Social Work in Palliative Care* published by the association and BASW in 2016.

Gillian Chowns is a social worker by profession, and has practised, lectured and researched in palliative care. Her PhD examined the experience of children living with the life-threatening illness of a parent. She is Chair of the Board of Trustees of Palliative Care Works, a charity offering education, training and mentoring in resource-poor settings.

Andrew Cooper is a Professor of Social Work at the Tavistock Centre, London, and University of East London, UK. Teaching, researching and promoting relationship-based and therapeutic social work has been central to his career.

Anne Cullen is Community Engagement Programme Lead at Princess Alice Hospice, UK. She is also a PhD student at the University of Hull, UK. Her research interests are palliative care and social work leadership.

Jason Davidson currently manages Supportive Care Services at the Marie Curie Hospice in London, UK. A registered social worker, he has worked for Marie Curie for the last two years. His research interests include social work and leadership within the context of palliative care and hospice care. He also has a special interest in the end-of-life care experiences of people with a learning disability and is currently the national chair of the PCPLD (Palliative Care for People with Learning Disabilities) Network.

Andrea Dechamps is a Patient and Family Support Director, St Wilfrid's Hospice, UK. Her research interests include psychosocial support at end of life and social work in palliative care. She has lectured internationally on psychosocial aspects of end-of-life care and has served as a trustee of a community bereavement service and the Natural Death Centre.

NOTES ON CONTRIBUTORS

Sally Paul is a Lecturer in the School of Social Work and Social Policy at the University of Strathclyde, UK. Her current practice and research interests are in bereavement and loss, end-of-life and palliative care, compassionate communities, participatory research methods and practice and service development.

Heather Richardson is Joint Chief Executive of St Christopher's Hospice, London, and Honorary Professor in Palliative Care at Lancaster University, UK. She is a nurse, and has held clinical, managerial and leadership roles in hospice/palliative care over the last thirty years. Her PhD focused on people's experience of day hospice.

Katharine Scanlan is a registered doctoral student (Tavistock/UEL) and a visiting lecturer at the Tavistock Clinic. Having qualified as a social worker in 1987, she is pursuing a long-standing interest in palliative and end-of-life care through her current research.

Sue Taplin is a Senior Lecturer in Social Work at the Faculty of Health, Social Care and Education, Anglia Ruskin University, UK. She holds an MA/PG diploma in Social Work from the University of Leicester, UK, and a doctorate in Social Work from the University of East Anglia, UK. She practised as a social worker and practice educator in hospice and palliative care before embarking on a career in social work education.

INTRODUCTION

Social Work Practice in End of Life Care

This special issue focuses on end of life — something we know will happen to everyone, as well as serving as a professional area of interest for many. We are two individuals, drawn from different professional backgrounds who have come together to think more about the experiences of dying and loss, and the care for people who are living with a terminal illness or who are bereaved, through the lens of social workers with a systemic perspective. Our editorial considers the various complexities we have encountered in the course of our learning and how these might be addressed in the future, drawing on the themes of this special issue.

One of the first areas of difficulty lies in the language and terminology used. What, for example, do we mean by 'end of life'? When does 'the end' begin? And is end of life care the same as ' palliative care'? What distinctions should be drawn between 'supportive care' and 'compassionate care' — or can all of these terms be used interchangeably? All professions, including academia, and health and social care, not only develop their own language and terminology, but, some would say, are also prey to changing fashions. When Dame Cicely Saunders first challenged the medical profession on the care of the dying, the phrase 'terminal care' was widely used. Connotations of negativity ('there is nothing more we can do,') finality and last resort led to the more favoured use of 'palliative care' and until relatively recently this has been the preferred term — care that is offered to those whose condition cannot be cured (from the Latin **pallium**, to cover, and thence, to ease or alleviate) — a phrase, however, that elicits no understanding from many people, be they lay or professional. A memorable experience, for one of the editors, was to introduce herself as 'from the palliative care team' at the Reception desk of a social work office and to be asked 'Oh, where's that?' as if it was the name of a parish or district.

It has been argued that this term has also reinforced the view that palliative care **follows on** from curative attempts, rather than running alongside, in tandem. Perhaps for this reason, 'supportive care' (offering support from diagnosis to death and, for the family, beyond into bereavement) has enjoyed a vogue in more recent years, although it has been justifiably critiqued on two counts: the vagueness of the word 'supportive', and the possible implication that any other care is not necessarily supportive. A similar criticism could be made of the currently popular term 'compassionate care'; broader, more readily comprehensible than 'palliative care' and more socially than medically focused, it nevertheless carries an element of preciousness — that compassion is the hallmark of our work that others do not achieve, or only to a lesser extent.

Currently, the World Health Organisation continues to use the term 'palliative care' and defines it as follows;

> Palliative care is an approach that improves the quality of life of patients and their families facing the problems associated with life-threatening illness, through the

prevention and relief of suffering by means of early identification and impeccable assessment and treatment of pain and other problems, physical, psychosocial and spiritual.

Clearly, a holistic approach is the foundation of such care, and even if we might critique the implicit arrogance of 'impeccable', social workers welcome the recognition of the importance of the psychosocial and spiritual, alongside the physical, in the WHO definition of palliative care.

Nevertheless, in contemporary debate, 'end-of life care' is frequently the phrase of choice. It can be argued that it is more inclusive than palliative care, where illness in general, and cancer in particular, has been the central focus. Palliation is inevitably associated with medicine, whereas 'end-of-life' sits more comfortably in public discourse and encompasses the social context more readily. In addition, its virtue of simplicity and clarity is immediately obvious — until one interrogates it further to define the point at which one's client, patient or family member is reaching the 'end'. In this issue the reader will encounter all these terms, sometimes used interchangeably. But terminology always matters; definitions shape policy and practice, and can subtly influence the 'reach' of our work, both enabling and embracing, but also excluding or ignoring. For example, for many decades, palliative care, if not synonymous with cancer, was certainly not available to those with dementia. Contemporary policy and practice recognizes that dementia is a major social problem in an ageing society and that those affected will need care which is supportive, compassionate, skilled and timely as their condition advances. To what degree professionals and services delivering palliative care see themselves as responsible for reaching out to people with dementia is currently variable, as organisations such as hospices consider their appropriateness to meeting such needs.

Then there is the complex interaction between the personal, individual, internal world of both patient and professional, on the one hand, and on the other, the tensions inherent in, and between organisations, systems, agencies and society itself. This clash, as it so often is, exists throughout all areas of social work, with both worker and client frequently finding themselves caught between systems designed to ensure equity and efficiency and, on the other hand, lived experiences which fail to fit neatly into prescribed boxes.

Another tension lies in the relative importance of addressing inadequacies of end of life care in a context of growing (and increasingly unmet) demands for health and social care. In the course of 2015, the Parliamentary and Health Service Ombudsman highlighted significant failures in the provision of NHS care for people at the end of life. Its report 'Dying without Dignity' suggests that the NHS needs to become better at recognizing that people are dying, making sure that symptoms are properly controlled, communicating with people, their families and each other, providing care around the clock, 365 days a year, and coordinating care better in response to people's needs. Just six months later, the Economist Intelligence Unit measured the quality of palliative care across 80 countries and confirmed that the UK ranked first. It suggests that the comprehensive national policies developed in this country, the extensive integration of palliative care into the NHS, a strong hospice movement and significant community engagement are major contributory factors. Then, in between the publication of these two significant and somewhat contradictory reports, the UK witnessed the second reading of a bill in the House of Commons to enable competent adults who are terminally ill to choose to be provided with medically supervised assistance to end their own life. Proponents of the bill described it as a piece of legislation called for by the vast majority of the public who wanted greater choice around when and how they died (Dignity in Dying Website). Those opposed to it, (for example the organisation Care not Killing) suggest that the vast majority of the public fear legalized assisted dying on behalf of people who may feel a burden to others in their illness and feel pressure to bring their life to a premature end; the same group also suggest that the public are concerned that NHS managers or politicians would prioritise assisted dying over end of life care to save money in the longer term. In the event, the bill was rejected. Regardless, issues of control and choice in terminal illness remain important for *many* individuals.

Finally, there is a question of what end of life care will need to look like in the future to meet changing needs. There is good evidence that the requirement for end of life care will increase significantly in the future and that the nature of these requirements will change. The UK and elsewhere are already witnessing an increase in the size of their populations and the numbers of people who are dying; this is a trend that is only likely to continue. In addition people are living much longer and dying at an older age. As a result people die differently from those who died twenty or thirty years ago. Most of us are most likely to die whilst suffering from more than one condition; in addition we may well have been living with a chronic illness for a number of years prior to death. We are increasingly likely to be living alone and our access to family carers will be radically reduced.

The articles in this special issue highlight some of the possible responses to this complex context.

Andrew Cooper offers a good place to start as he explores a number of contemporary perspectives on the nature of a good death. His thoughts are drawn from his personal experience, and that of others — including one of the other authors — Katharine Scanlan, quite by chance. We are drawn to his candid descriptions of connection and disconnection, presence and loss in the processes of dying and bereavement, and of his suggestion of the opportunity of 'an afterlife' by being held in the minds of others. The paper serves to remind us that death is utterly personal — it happens to individuals, interrupts vital relationships and leaves an imprint in the thoughts of those who survive. The way to experience a good death is, he suggests, by engagement in the challenging psychological interactions between the living and the dying.

Then, there is the call for communication, communication, communication. As both Becky Chaddock and, later, Lesley Adshead and Andrea Deschamps aver, this is the bedrock of both social work in general and palliative care social work in particular. While Chaddock sets out a Cumbrian strategy on Advance Directives — with its attendant systems, and standard forms — for enabling end of life discussions to happen in a range of settings, she makes the point strongly that it is the quality of the conversations that is paramount, and not the completion of the paperwork. Similarly, in reflecting on their innovative partnerships with local authorities, Adshead and Deschamps acknowledge that many of the local authority social workers that they have trained already possess good communication skills 'but lack the confidence to fully utilise them in relation to end of life'.

Another thread — clearly connected to skilled communication — is that of containment, a familiar concept for readers of this journal. In Katharine Scanlan's thoughtful application of psychoanalytical understandings to the practice, and patient and family experience, of palliative care, she explores a 'third way' in which professionals, organisations and individuals can contain the inevitable fear and pain associated with death and dying. Such fear and pain is not, however, the exclusive preserve of those whose life is close to its end, as Sue Taplin reminds us. Her exploration of cancer 'survivors' — those who live to tell the tale — is a timely reminder that this is a growing, though often neglected, group who live, but live in a state of liminality and ambivalence. For some of them, though not all, incorporating their illness into a new 'normal' lifestyle was the preferred way to contain both the illness and its associated dynamics.

Alongside communication and containment, the importance of community emerges as a significant and sometimes contested thread. Although Scanlan's and Taplin's papers focus on the psychodynamic aspects of living through and dying of cancer, they nevertheless both acknowledge the social and organizational settings in which the experience is embedded. End of life care can never be exclusively the province of health care. As Lesley Adshead and Andrea Deschamps claim, it is everybody's business; life and death, are, in the widest sense, social events. This reframe of dying, in a context of community has been the subject of a number of writers in recent years, who promote an alternative approach to end of life care, that of new public health. In so doing, they critique what they see as a preciosity on the part of many hospices and palliative care services to claim end of life care as the almost exclusive domain of professionals. In doing so, they have served to disempower both families and communities. This is a serious charge and one which Adshead and De Champs largely refute in their careful analysis of Walter and Brown's critique of current practice. These authors then go on to reflect on their own experience of collaborating with local authority staff and others to offer a community oriented training and working partnership, which acknowledges and builds on the strengths of those outwith the traditional hospice and palliative care settings.

The recent emphasis on public health approaches, including compassionate communities, to end of life is therefore to be warmly welcomed in our view and must be embraced by social workers. Its approach, which focuses on equity, participation and a broader understanding of health and wellbeing, is consistent with the values of social work. Sally Paul writes convincingly of the role of the social worker in identifying and supporting community responses to bereavement and loss in schools, and of the potential interest, energy and innovation that lies therein. Jason Davidson confirms it as an important opportunity in which social workers could offer a leadership role. Chaddock's article demonstrates how a genuinely collaborative approach, involving mainstream health and social care organisations from first ideas to full inception, can contribute to greater awareness and understanding, and therefore better decision-making not just by specialized professionals but throughout wider society, and echoes this theme.

Enabling people to find meaning in the course of a life threatening illness or in bereavement is another thread. The International Federation of Social Workers' (IFSW) definition of social work requires workers, inter alia, to promote 'the empowerment and liberation of people' and to engage 'people and structures to address life challenges and enhance wellbeing'. Readers of this journal will immediately appreciate the relevance of the role of the social worker in ensuring that good psychosocial care remains an integral part of the service offered to the seriously ill and dying, and to their families. A systemic perspective respects the importance of context, the power of the individual's inner world, the existential threat posed by the approach of death and the primacy of relationships in giving meaning to both the client's living and their dying.

Both Scanlan and Taplin focus on this process of meaning-making. Scanlan's article highlights the way in which some professionals lack insight into both their own and their patients' and clients' internal worlds, and offers a model for understanding the complex dynamics that occur so often as individuals struggle to contain their fears of mortality. While Scanlan draws on a combination of her own personal experience allied to her training in psychodynamic social work, to examine the internal processes that can make or mar the care that is offered, Taplin investigates the experience of those whose cancer diagnosis has not proved 'terminal' — the survivors. For many individuals, while finishing treatment is not an unalloyed pleasure, as they can feel as if they have been set adrift and abandoned by their professional carers, survivorship undoubtedly leads to a re-ordering of their assumptive world. Taplin identifies several significant themes that emerge from her research with this sometimes marginalized group.

A requirement to change the way we think about, organise and deliver end of life care is the final thread. There are clear indicators that we must move to a more integrated model of care — encompassing health and social care, along with more support and education for family carers, neighbours and friends if we are to meet changing needs and preferences. New models of care call for different models of leadership. Davidson confirms that social workers must be leaders in the future. However, his research confirms that this will require significant cultural change and training if social workers are to be enabled to step up to this mark. We will also need to think differently about how we support staff to deliver the kind of care that is required in the future. Our experience in practice suggests that nurses, doctors, social workers and others are already struggling to meet existing demands. How do we build their resilience and that of the organisations that must lead and deliver end of life care to more people with more complex needs, particularly given the evidence that compassionate care is linked closely to staff who feel supported in their work? New approaches such as Schwartz rounds are being established and evaluated in the UK. Ann Cullen makes a strong case for this approach in building the emotional resilience of staff engaged in end of life care and the role of social workers in supporting this initiative.

As we conclude, we reflect on the role of the social worker in end of life care and the potential application of the themes arising from these papers, for social workers who do not work with people who are dying or bereaved, but who nevertheless are always working with loss in one form or another. In working with those facing the end of their own, or a family member's life, palliative care social workers draw on the same range of skills as those in local authority, hospital, mental health and other settings, as Chaddock makes clear in her article on Advance Directives. However in end of life care they are delivered in a specific context of (generally) very limited time, no prior experience (of one's own dying) upon which to draw, and a culture that, even in the twenty-first century, struggles to confront, and communicate openly about, death and dying. This makes the task just as, and sometimes more, challenging than that of social workers in other settings. Regardless, the core skills in all settings are honest, empathic communication, an ability to go beyond the spoken word and explore the inner world of the client, and to engage with both the family and the social context. We hope that this set of papers encourages readers to continue to hone these skills drawing on the evidence base provided by the papers, and that where social workers are working in end of life care, they will be encouraged to seek ways to strengthen their contribution to leadership issues, resilience and community participation in care, confident of the value of a social response to dying.

Gillian Chowns

Heather Richardson

Andrew Cooper

A GOOD DEATH?

'It frightens me the awful truth of how sweet life can be' Bob Dylan

This paper offers some personal reflections on the idea of 'a good death', a theme in the writing of philosophers since classical times. The hospice movement has made immense progress in creating conditions in which we can 'die better'. But such experiences are still the exception rather than the rule. The psychological challenge is how to relate to the dying as they are dying, and how as we die we relate to the living. I reflect on my own experience of my father's death, and a moment of fleeting but genuine contact between us. Atul Gawande's idea of the 'hard conversations' we must learn to have as we approach death are enlightening. Ultimately I argue, we die alone, and how we are, or are not, 'held in mind' as we approach death may be an index of the nearest we can approach to the idea of an 'afterlife'.

A great place to die?

'I wish I could tell people how nice it can be to die of cancer.' This is the first line of Colin Murray Parkes' foreword to Elisabeth Kubler-Ross's classic (1969) text *On Death and Dying*. He is quoting a woman who died peacefully in a Hospice a few days later. '"Can be" — but, too often, is not', Murray Parkes adds a few lines later.

The UK is now officially the best country in the world in which to die, according to the 2015 Quality of Death Index (EIU, 2015) which ranks palliative care across the globe. Indeed with a score of 93.9 out of 100, it can't get that much better. Iraq with a score of 12.5 props up the list of 80 countries surveyed. I am sure the irony of this will not be lost on readers, though it is not a point on which I want to dwell. The UK picture probably ought to provide us with some reassurance, as we contemplate more directly our own relationship to dying, which is part of what I want to help us do in this paper. But I wonder how much comfort it really does offer?

The hospice and palliative care movement in this country, and globally, have positively transformed our social capacity to think about dying and death as a part of life, and to create circumstances in which tens of thousands of people undoubtedly have been able to die better than was once possible. Rereading Kubler-Ross's book after 30 years was a daunting experience. What could I possibly add to the wisdom and humanity of this moving and profoundly insightful work? And yet, I think there is more to say.

The model of a good death which this work has generated, of last weeks, days and hours attended by thoughtful and experienced professionals able to tolerate and think about intense emotional pain, help those close to the dying person achieve something of the same, while physical pain is also skillfully moderated — this it seems to me remains an experience available only to a few, and not only because of the limited resources we have to offer such care. The danger is that we idealise this rather privileged notion of 'a good death' and take false comfort from our unfamiliar position at the top of this league table.

Death is not an event in life — or is it?

The inquiry into Mid Staffordshire NHS hospital trust, the Francis Report (2010) exposed standards of care for the ill and the dying that seem truly appalling, but which I suspect surprised fewer of us than it shocked. Anyone who in recent years has been an inpatient in a hard pressed general hospital might have some inkling of how and why matters could deteriorate to the degree that was revealed by Francis. But the mystery of how and why so much neglect, insensitivity and even cruelty, could become routine and normalized has not been solved, at least not to my satisfaction. The solution is obviously complex, and I mainly want to address just one dimension in what follows.

In summary, our relationship to death poses us with an extreme instance of something more general and familiar to anyone who works in the field of mental health or social care, namely how hard it is emotionally to keep moving towards rather than away from intense mental pain and anxiety, and how correspondingly hard it is to create and maintain organizational systems that support this simple but exceptionally challenging task.

The philosopher Ludwig Wittgenstein once wrote, 'Death is not an event in life: we do not live to experience death'(Wittgenstein, 1972). This seems right, and I suggest most of us are terrified of death because we do not want to stop living, not because we fear what lies beyond death. But of course death is an 'event in life' for all those left behind, and so the idea of a good death is, I suggest, all about how to live in relation to others *as we are dying* and how those of us close to the dying live and relate to the dying *as they are dying*. Perhaps the phrase 'a good death' subtly shields us from this, to me more challenging but also realistic formulation. Also, the question arises 'for whom is a good death good?', the dying person or those attending, and destined to survive, and can the one find accommodation with the other?

As I prepared this paper, it gradually dawned on me that there are just so many ways to die, and also so many ways in which our own mortality, and that of others, may impinge on us during the course of life. Another philosopher, Spinoza, wrote that 'A free man thinks of nothing less than of death, and his wisdom is a meditation upon life, not upon death' (Spinoza, 1930). In my early twenties I wrote a long post-graduate thesis about Spinoza, and inscribed this quote on the cover of a green A4 notebook I kept. During this period I was also ill with Hodgkins Disease, a life threatening but even in those days treatable cancer of the lymphatic system. I survived, and indeed also survived a recurrence a few years later. I still think Spinoza's words are wise, but I also presume it was no accident that I selected this proposition from his *Ethics* rather any number of other choice observations, for my notebook cover. Death and dying were very much on my mind, whatever reassurances I was receiving about my prognosis. My first published paper, in the *Lancet*, was an account of my experiences as a Hodgkins patient, and I wrote there that 'To the oncologist a 90% survival rate may look pretty impressive. To me as a patient it looked more like a one in ten chance of dying very soon' (Cooper, 1982).

Sooner or later then, death, our own mortality, forces itself upon our attention. I was unfortunate to have to wrestle with this so young, but eventually nearly all of us will confront this state of affairs. The exceptions, I suppose, include those of us who drop suddenly and unexpectedly dead from a brain hemorrhage or heart attack, or similar—it happened to my young son's football coach, a vigorous, energetic man in his mid-40s, and to my own older brother when he was 58. A few among us may die suddenly and violently in road accidents, plane crashes, terrorist attacks and the like, but a greater proportion of us will die after suffering a lengthy dementia of some kind that will rob us of most of our psychological agency in relation to our dying.

'Cold, stone coloured, like marble…'

For all these reasons, and more, the question mark in the title of this paper became for me its focal point. So I want to borrow from one personal experience of a very different kind of death, to remind us that for many death and dying just does remains unpredictable, uncontrollable, and unthinkably painful.

Some years after the death of her 19 month old son Joe, Denise Turner carried out systematic qualitative research with parents who had experienced sudden, unexpected infant death. Her own experience, skillfully and sensitively mediated, lies at the emotional root of this work, and of her own researcher sensitivity, and here she tells the story of finding her son dead. Joe was one of twins, born prematurely, and he had always been vulnerable to colds and chest infections but Denise had been reassured that this was nothing serious.

> One Sunday night in March 2005 Joe seemed a bit snuffly. I took his temperature which was normal, checked for signs of a rash and reassured put him to bed as usual. He drank a good bottle of bedtime milk. Colds were very common and because I had been told Joe was a 'Happy Wheezer', I was not unduly concerned.

> In the morning, Amy came into bed with me before I went downstairs to get the boys their milk; she went in to say good morning to them. When I walked into the room a few moments later, she was sitting in Dan's cot reading to him. Joe was lying face down in his own cot. 'Joe's still asleep Mummy' she said. I took one look at him. He was cold, stone coloured, like marble. I knew immediately that he had been dead for hours. The moment is frozen in my mind like a still from a film. It is one of those moments that perhaps most parents rehearse in their heads, hoping it will never happen and wondering what they will do if it does? What I did was

to get Amy and Dan out of the room. Joe was dead. There was nothing I could do for him. My instinct, in that second was for my two living children. 'Yes,' I said, 'Joe's still asleep. Let's not disturb him.' And I settled them downstairs (Turner, 2013, pp. 26–27).

A central theme of Denise Turner's research is the impact on parents and other family members of the policy led professional response to a death of this kind, known as a rapid response protocol. Almost within minutes of alerting services, her home became a crime scene, swarming with professionals, and the body of her son became the legal property of the coroner.

'Part of me anticipated the moment of my arrest and the removal of my two surviving children. Like Davies (2010, p. 7) I felt 'undermined, disbelieved and threatened', propelled by random tragedy into a world of police investigation and forensic evidence where I was a suspect in my own home, only minutes after finding my son dead in his cot (2013, p. 29).

Later she reflects

…one of my lasting impressions of Joe's death (is that)… most of the professionals involved were having a terrible time. No one seemed genuinely able to cope. The horror of the situation, the fear of being held culpable and the sheer randomness of the death seemed to immobilize people's basic humanity at this most human of times (2013, p. 32).

Implicitly, she links these observations to what subsequently ensued

What did surprise me (however) was that hardly anyone came. The G.P. called briefly that night to check on Dan. After the tidal wave of professionals who filled our home that morning had dispersed, we were left in the weeks that followed to cope with our two surviving children; the shock of Joe's death and the surrounding events, as well as the countless tasks that follow a death, with almost no support (2013, p. 30).

Dying in twenty-first Century Britain

This story points up certain paradoxes about death and dying in twenty-first century Britain. Concurrent with the progress we have made in creating authentically responsive and caring spaces and places in which to negotiate dying and death, we have also bureaucratized, proceduralised and protocolised death. Controversies over the so called Liverpool End of Life Care Pathway are a manifestation of this tension. This reflects the experience of mental health and social care works more generally, that they aspire all the time to work in close relationship with people, but find themselves constrained by the requirements of statute, policy, procedure, guidance, protocol and performance management regimes to operate in a perfunctory manner that meets organizational needs but neglects the lived experience of service users. It is too simple to explain this bureaucratizing trend as a just another variety of 'social defence' against the anxieties of death and dying or other forms of mental pain, the organizational normalization of professional practices that distance people from the pain of the work, as described by Menzies Lyth in her classic paper about general nurses in a general hospital (Lyth, 1959). But Denise Turner's experience of immediate, intense, but also institutionally suspicious professional responses succeeded by prolonged neglect of her emotional circumstances suggests a dynamic in which we may move towards dying and death when compelled to do so, but too often in a spirit of anxious mistrust, only then to flee the scene leaving the bereaved entirely 'dropped from mind'. While perfunctory and routinized responses to the lived experience of a dying or bereaved person may be conveniently and unhelpfully *supported* by organizational cultures of procedure and risk aversion, such responses will emanate as much from our own deep anxiety about how to really 'be with', or stay alongside, people traversing dying and death.

My father, his father, and me

So also when I was in my in my twenties, my father died after a long dementing illness. I had a lot of difficulty communicating and relating to him through this period, as did all his family I think, and he was not a man who was ever comfortable with strong feelings or emotional pain. But one evening as I sat quietly and anxiously with him he suddenly said to me, 'I wish I could die like my father did. He sat down after lunch one day, had a heart attack and died just like that'. It was the most poignant and painful communication my father ever made to me. In the midst of his suffering and disorientation, I think my grandfather's death became my father's idea of a good death. I cannot be sure, but I now suspect that my father was just appallingly lonely during these last years, exactly because no one around him could bear, or could summon the emotional resources, to find a way to come closer to him.

The sociologist Clive Seale speaks of dying people 'falling from culture' (Seale, 1998) as they become more dependent and unwell in the period, sometimes lengthy, that precedes death, as they lose connection with the networks and routine relationships that are the taken for granted social tissue of our aliveness. Thus what he calls 'social death' may often precede the death of the body. It is family and perhaps close friends who are there, or not, to accompany the dying person in their final period of life, and a disproportionate burden of this task falls of course to women. The emotional task of truly 'being with' someone as they approach their death, so that they do not experience themselves as 'dropped from mind' by those closest to them, is perhaps one of the greatest tests of emotional maturity that any of us will face.

I felt hopelessly inadequate in the face of my father's process of dying, and guilty for many years afterwards. Eventually it was a relief to let go of any ambivalence I felt towards him as my father, and say to myself, 'I wish I had been able to be a better son to you'. But in writing this paper, I came to a slightly different view of matters. His communication to me, and my receipt of it, was not nothing. Out of the silence, the void that I remember him apparently inhabiting much of the time as he deteriorated, he *was* able to formulate this expression of his distress, in effect of his wish to die and be released, and deliver it to me. And I was at least there to receive it. There could have been so much more, but I suspect that even such a fleeting moment of connection as this is hard won by all involved. Maybe there were other moments with my mother or other family members, I don't know. We just didn't talk properly about it. But I offer this story, and these thoughts, to provide us with some sense of the difficulties that face us as we try to think well about this idea of 'relating to dying' — what we might hope for as we ourselves approach death, and what we might hope for from ourselves in relating to others in their dying. And finally, recognizing the depth of the emotional challenge involved, the value of forgiveness for what we fail to achieve with others, or to receive from them.

This is the territory explored by Gawande (2014) in his profound and important book *Being Mortal: Illness, Medicine and What Matters in the End'*. In the space that lies between manic hope or denial, and helpless resignation in the face of the knowledge of imminent death, Gawande describes the 'hard conversations' the dying and the living need to have, so that the dying person can exercise maximum feasible choice about how they spend their last weeks, days and hours. Medicine has become heroically addicted to prolonging life at all costs, disabling everyone's ability to weigh the balance between longevity and quality of life in the final phases of living. 'Assisted living is far harder that assisted death', writes Gawande, 'but its possibilities are far greater as well'. Our ultimate goal, after all, is not a good death but a good life to the very end' (2014, p. 245).

Beyond death

Some people and families do manage what we might all think of as a good death, or a good life to the very end. I have witnessed it and I expect many readers have as well. If I have dwelt on the challenges and impediments to dying well then that is because I suspect that 'good deaths' remain the exception rather than the rule, even in our supposedly advanced society. There is a school of thought and practice, best represented maybe by the British Humanist Society, that tries to approach death and dying rationally, free from illusions about an afterlife or salvation of the soul, but nevertheless deeply respectful of our need for meaning in relation to death and loss. I think Spinoza's stance — cited above - is consistent with this ethos. Death and dying take their meaning from life, and the deep mourning that attends the loss of life, whether imminent or actual. The terror of this loss, the ultimate loss, at once evoking and transcending all other losses we have experienced, is what renders dying so hard to bear.

I think the existential reality is that we each die alone. No one can do it for us, and no one can accompany us in death itself, only on our passage towards it, or if we are the survivor, following it. But this is not the same as dying in a state of loneliness. In a secular way of thinking, our salvation, our after life if you prefer, resides in the possibility of being remembered and held in the minds of others long after death. In this respect I offer another short extract from the autobiographical writing of another researcher into modern experiences of dying. Here she is recalling her father's death.

On the night he died I was at home with my children. My husband was out and the friend I had spent the evening with talking about my father, stayed so that I could go by taxi to my parent's home within a few minutes of his death. When I arrived I was able to help my mother wash him and get him ready to leave his home for the last time. It is difficult to fully describe just how much being able to perform this ritual meant to us both. It was at the time, and remains now, one of the most significant things I have ever done. It felt completely right and appropriate, and something that we could do for him before we had to let him go. It was a way of beginning to love him beyond life (Scanlan, 2014, pers. commun.).

To know, or to echo the Christian form of words, 'to have a sure and certain hope' that we might be loved, remembered and cared for in our afterlife in such a manner might be the nearest we can approach to answering the probably universal need for a 'good death' — that which we all hope for, but may or may not be granted.

Disclosure statement

No potential conflict of interest was reported by the authors.

References

Cooper, A. (1982) 'Disabilities and how to live with them: Hodgkin's disease', *The Lancet*, vol. 1, no. 8272, pp. 612–613.

Economics Intelligence Unit. (2015) 'The 2015 quality of death index. Ranking palliative care across the world'. EIU, London.

Francis, R. (2010) *Independent Inquiry into Care Provided by Mid Staffordshire NHS Foundation Trust: January 2005–March 2009* (Vol. 375), The Stationery Office, London.

Gawande, A. (2014) *Being Mortal: Medicine and What Matters in the End*, Macmillan, London.

Kubler-Ross, E. (1969) *On Death and Dying*, Macmillan Publishing, New York, NY.

Menzies Lyth, I. M. (1959) 'The functions of social systems as a defence against anxiety: a report on a study of the nursing service of a general hospital', *Human Relations*, vol. 13, pp. 95–121.

Seale, C. (1998) *Constructing Death*, Cambridge University Press, Cambridge.

Spinoza, B. (1930) 'The Ethics', In *Spinoza, Selections*, ed. J. Wild. Charles Scribners Sons, New York, pp. 346.

Turner, D. (2013) *Telling the Story: What can be Learned from Parents' Experience of the Professional Response Following the Sudden, Unexpected Death of a Child*. [Unpublished PhD thesis], University of Sussex, Brighton.

Wittgenstein, L. (1972) *Tractatus Logico-Philosophicus*, Routledge & Kegan Paul, London.

Katharine Scanlan

PSYCHOSOCIAL PERSPECTIVES ON END OF LIFE CARE

Personal and professional experience has made the author aware of the way in which emotional responses to vulnerability, life threatening illness, death and dying can significantly influence the course and outcome of medical and social interventions, as well as the provision and quality of care provided. In recent years psychoanalytic studies have enabled a deeper understanding of the unconscious primitive anxieties and associated defences that are part of being human, and to think about the implications for health and social care workers as society strives to meet the needs of an increasingly ageing population. Aspects of psychoanalytic theory, including contemporary applications, have been useful in reflecting on what it means to provide care for those at the end of life. The author will discuss the value of applying psychoanalytic understanding and faculties to this developing area of health and social care. Early findings from a doctoral research project, "Bringing Death Home", will be referred to. The conclusion will reflect on personal knowledge and lived experience of palliative care social work to consider the significant contribution that relationship-based social work practice can make to the ongoing implementation of the end of life care strategy and the wider integrated care agenda.

Introduction

There is evidence to suggest that significant attempts are being made to examine and reshape society's relationship with death, dying and end of life. The reasons for this growing awareness of, and concern about, what has in recent years become a somewhat neglected and 'split-off' aspect of human experience are perhaps not too difficult to understand. Statistics provide a useful starting point and an Age UK briefing summary published in 2014 highlights the fact that the number of people aged eight-five years or over has increased by 30 per cent in the years between 2005 and 2014. The focus of this particular report is funding for social care, or perhaps at the present time, the lack of it, but as such it provides considerable insight in to what it means to grow old and reach the end of life in the early years of the twenty-first century. There is a sense that we have reached a point in our evolution as a society that we have not fully prepared for and that many of us had, and perhaps still do, hope to avoid for as long as possible. The figures given by the Age UK report make it clear that this is no longer possible and that difficult and potentially painful decisions must be made if the end of life care needs of an ageing population are to be met.

The place that death and dying has come to occupy and that recent strategies and movements are working so hard to amend has come about over time and as a result of complex factors including the scientific and technological advances that have determined how we organize our private lives. The history of our relationship with death in the Western world is well documented with a number of writers telling a similar story from a range of perspectives (Aries, 1982; Walter, 1994; Holloway, 2007). An overview of a number of these accounts suggests that at least since the beginning of the previous century people living in the Western world have become less familiar with death and that the end of life has increasingly become the domain of health care professionals.

As a result, some of the issues emerging in recent years have included the unnecessary prolongation of life often through invasive and potentially traumatic interventions and the inappropriateness of hospitals as places to be cared for at the end of life. The Liverpool Care Pathway (LCP), an early attempt to provide guidance to those caring at the end of life, was often misinterpreted and subsequently abandoned. Similarly the right of individuals to choose to die has been debated and contested leaving those wishing to end their lives to make the necessary arrangements whilst still well enough to do so.

The hospice movement and palliative care are recognized as having the specialist skills and knowledge to lead the way and since the implementation of the End of Life Care Strategy (2008) it is clear that more people are dying at home or in their preferred place of care. Individuals and communities are being encouraged and supported to talk about death and dying and end of life care is firmly on the agenda in health and social care and a primary concern in the integration of services. However, when it comes to the experience of close personal care and the management of individual cases it seems that the strategies and best intentions of the organizations promoting compassionate end of life care for all can be undermined sometimes subtly but often in thoughtless, and at times even cruel, ways.

Despite a proliferation of quality standards (NICE, 2011/2013) and guidance (Leadership Alliance for the Care of Dying People 2014) recent reports suggest that the kind of care people want at the end of life (Dying Well Community Charter, 2014) is not always easy to achieve or sustain. A recent report of investigations into complaints about end of life care by the Parliamentary and Health Service Ombudsman (2015) concludes 'there is a need for the NHS to get better' in a number of areas of end of life care including recognizing that people are dying, and communicating openly yet sensitively with people, their families and each other about care towards the end of life. Earlier in 2014 an NCP report noted that the review of the LCP in 2013 recognized that 'whilst many people who died on the LCP received good care, that there were also far too many cases of people who had been treated poorly, both those at the end of life and their families'.

This paper is an attempt to reach a deeper understanding of the complexities of caring for those at the end of life and to consider what might help support the kind of systems of care that can respond to the challenge.

An ongoing relationship

When my father became ill in the spring of 1984 I was twenty-seven years old with two small children aged just four and eighteen months. Our family was deeply shocked; we seemed wholly unprepared for the possibility of life threatening illness and it took a while before we were able to comprehend and respond to the events that unfolded in a relatively short time period.

Although I had experienced the loss of three grandparents by this age my youth, my parents and my lack of experience, had all protected me from the full emotional impact. My paternal grandmother died suddenly from a heart attack, as did my maternal grandfather. Both deaths whilst shocking seemed complete and unambiguous. Later when my paternal grandfather became seriously ill and was taken to hospital I felt troubled when I visited him after his admission, by his account of being resuscitated. From his description I understood that he had experienced this as traumatic and when he died soon after in the same hospital felt a deep sense of regret that his life had ended this way. During his life we had connected deeply and I wonder now if this is when I first became aware of the significance of end of life care and the importance of 'getting it right' for the individual concerned (One Chance To Get It Right, LADP, 2014).

Certainly when it became apparent that my father was reaching the end of his life with an aggressive and untreatable cancer I found myself acutely attuned to his needs and appalled by what seemed to be an uncaring and at times deliberately cruel health service. I will never forget my father's face when presented with a lunch menu and asked to choose his lunch. This seemed a particularly thoughtless way to care for a man who had been admitted because of his increasing inability to swallow anything remotely solid.

In this and countless other ways the health system appeared unable to respond appropriately and the care he received seemed to be represented by the kind of things I later found had been identified by Menzies Lyth in her study of the nursing service in a London hospital practice as far back as 1959 (Menzies, 1960). The defensive techniques she discovered at that time included depersonalization, categorisation, detachment and denial of feelings. This was my first experience of personal and organizational defence mechanisms and of their impact on all concerned. In subsequent years they have become more familiar and increasingly central to my thinking on end of life matters. I have come to understand defences as necessary and protective as well as potentially pathological and disorientating (Kubler-Ross, 1969, p. 20). As my father reached the end of his life they were represented in all of these forms.

Lacking a theoretical framework to make sense of what was occurring I muddled through in an intuitive, instinctive, kind of way. Desperate to remove him to a safe place a close friend of my sister's who had trained as a nurse agreed to come and stay in my parent's home and oversee his care during the final stages of his illness. Although we knew her offer was precious it is only now that I fully understand its significance as a potential model of end of life care in 2015. Without her involvement and support I am almost certain that my father would have been unable to remain at home. As it was, the various crises including an intense period of agitation were managed well and he died peacefully in his own bed.

There is no doubt that my professional interest in and commitment to palliative care and the work of the hospice movement (Saunders, 1990) has personal origins. Following my father's death I qualified as a social worker, completing my final placement in our recently opened local hospice, where I found myself in an environment engaged in enabling those with a life limiting illness to live as fully as possible and to die with dignity. The foundations of my knowledge and understanding of loss and grief, of the impact of living with a life limiting condition, and of the importance of holistic assessment and care were firmly established here and have influenced my personal and professional life profoundly ever since.

Later when I returned to the same hospice to manage the social work team and other psychosocial services I inherited a mature and committed staff team focused on the primary task of supporting patients, their families and significant others through some of the most challenging of human experiences. My theoretical framework included the work of Bowlby (1969, 1973,1980), Kubler-Ross (1969), Murray-Parkes (1998) and Worden (1991) as well as the work of Cicely Saunders (1990) the founder of the modern hospice movement, and Frances Sheldon (1997) one of the first palliative care social workers. Familiar with existing models of social work supervision I came to more fully understand that a significant aspect of my role involved emotionally supporting the social work team, bereavement volunteers, and other members of staff working directly with patients in the community.

The decision to leave the hospice in 1999 was at least partly prompted by my husband's feeling that my emotional energy would be better focused on the needs of our young family, although in retrospect I wonder if he felt that it brought death too close for comfort. By the time he became ill in 2006 I had become used to thinking about death and dying from a distance and in a more abstract way. Although a close friend's husband had died a few years earlier it had not occurred to me that the same thing would happen to us and I was shocked to find that I was living with dying in the most intimate way possible.

Despite my knowledge and experience and possibly even because of it I denied what was happening for as long as possible — as did my husband. We hoped for a different outcome and wanted to avoid what turned out to be inevitable until the last possible moment. An early misdiagnosis contributed to the general confusion and a late terminal diagnosis was couched in terms of 'take him home and have a family barbecue with fine wine'. Our children were aged twelve and seventeen and our life together was coming to an end. When my husband arrived home able to breathe only with the help of huge oxygen generators that became the heartbeat of our house, and with a bottle of liquid morphine, I finally came to realise that we needed appropriate help if we were to manage the end of his life in any kind of bearable way.

Overwhelmed by primitive anxiety and in the grip of unconscious drives I found that I had retained some capacity for reflective thought and for what I have since learned and developed further, an internal professional structure or third position (Bower, 2003).

When my husband was eventually admitted to the hospice he received the physical care he desperately needed and the reassurance that everything would be done to make him as comfortable as possible. A hospice social worker focused on the needs of the children and arranged for us to spend as much time at the hospice as possible. For the first time during the course of his illness someone — a hospice doctor with many years' experience — spent time with us and gently but firmly acknowledged the seriousness of the situation. The same doctor met with myself, and our two children to explain that their father would not get better and had only a short time left to live. These interventions allowed us to find some way to respond to the reality of what was occurring and to organize ourselves in order to be there for him at the end of his life.

Less than two years later and as I became increasingly concerned about my mother's health I enrolled for a Master's Degree in Psychoanalytic Studies having decided that this would allow me to extend my existing knowledge and engage more fully with the unconscious aspects of human experience. The start of my studies coincided with the devastating news that my mother's ever growing range of symptoms constituted a diagnosis of Motor Neurone Disease. More than twenty years after the death of my father, and in a different set of circumstances, I had the same sense of systems of care and the individuals representing them, struggling to respond to someone with a terminal diagnosis and facing the end of life. Acutely sensitive to her needs and prompted by a particularly obscure and difficult 'do not resuscitate' conversation with a hospital registrar, I recognized ahead of the specialist MND nurse, that my mother was reaching the end of her life and a subsequent admission to the hospice meant that she was comforted and reassured during her final days.

The similarities between professional and organizational responses to these experiences of living with dying, observed over a significant period of time, strongly suggested the value of gaining a deeper understanding of the forces at work. Behaviour, that at a conscious, rational, level seems difficult to comprehend, yet continues to have a direct impact on the quality of the care provided at end of life, is significant and worthy of attention. The themes emerging in my personal end of life experiences, in 1984 (my father), 2006 (my husband), and 2008 (my mother), chime with the findings of the latest Parliamentary and Health Service Ombudsman's (2015) investigations into complaints about end of life care. They include health care professionals failing to recognise that people are dying, failing to respond to the needs of those concerned and difficulties in communicating appropriately. The ongoing nature of these issues indicates that more is required beyond information about what people want and what professionals should do if better end of life care is to become more widely and consistently available.

Psychoanalytic perspectives on end of life care

A closer engagement with psychoanalytic knowledge has allowed connections to be made between apparently discrete yet closely related theories and to learn from personal and professional experiences of end of life care. Deep connections are apparent between established theories of attachment, separation and loss and object relations, making it possible to understand just how much Klein influenced Bowlby and to recognize the similarities between some of their concepts. The influence of psychoanalysis permeates Bowlby's work with Parkes' on the development of an attachment model of bereavement providing the foundations for Parkes' phases of grief (1998), and his thinking on traumatic loss connects directly with the psychoanalytic concept of transference (Freud, 1920) in his theory of the assumptive world.

Their theories represent something of a family tree of interrelated ideas that extend understanding of the conscious and unconscious emotional aspects of human relationships and their significance in shaping our experiences from the moment of our conception to the end of life. Klein's theoretical developments in relation to the inner world, including her discovery of the paranoid schizoid and depressive positions, are as relevant to end of life as to all aspects of human development. The concept of the paranoid schizoid and depressive positions as states of mind as well as developmental phases is particularly helpful in understanding the ways that people cope with anxiety throughout life and in times of extreme emotional distress.

States of mind are not determined by chronological age but by the developmental progress an individual has made over the course of their life and within the context of their emotional environment. For example, an adult may be in a state of mind that represents a much earlier stage of development. Indeed faced with a threat to our own survival or that of a significant other on whom we depend emotionally we all have the capacity to return to a much earlier paranoid schizoid state of mind if only temporarily.

Each position has a defining set of anxieties, defences against these anxieties and a particular way of object relating. From the paranoid schizoid position anxieties are about personal survival and the possibility of being destroyed, annihilated or simply no longer existing. This anxiety may result internally through the inner workings of the death instinct or in response to external conditions such as serious and potentially life threatening illness or other painful or traumatic life events. Paranoid schizoid defences include denial, splitting, projection, identification, idealization and omnipotence. The depressive position represents a developmental shift in which the object is recognized as a whole person who can be both hated and loved. Anxieties are about the survival of the object with defences represented by ambivalence and depressive anxiety such as guilt, concern and reparation.

Whether the defences associated with each position organize themselves in a healthy or pathological way will depend on the degree of anxiety involved, the resources available and the unique life experiences and history of each individual. What we do know is that faced with intolerable levels of anxiety we employ whatever defences will allow us to maintain our mental/psychic equilibrium, that we all use defences to protect ourselves from psychic pain and that we oscillate between these two positions throughout our lives (Budd and Rusbridger, 2005, p. 13).

Theories of loss and grief connect directly with psychodynamic thinking about social systems as defences against anxiety in Parkes' concept of the assumptive world. Introducing a collection of writing that offers a number of different perspectives on the concept, Kauffman describes the assumptive world as 'constituted by the psychological act of believing' (2002, p. 2). For Parkes, the assumptive world consists of constant internal constructs that support the ability to believe or assume things about the external world. It is these beliefs and assumptions that (at best) allow us to feel safe and secure, to anticipate the future with hope and a degree of certainty and to trust in the goodness of ourselves, and others.

Assumptive worlds are deeply personal but also shaped by shared beliefs as well as primitive fears and anxieties. According to Parkes, it is 'the life events that bring us face to face with the fact that our existing assumptive world can no longer keep us safe that are the most difficult to negotiate' (Parkes in Kauffman, 2003, p. 238). The loss or anticipated loss of our assumptive world has the potential to breach our psychic defences, fears and anxieties are uncontained creating the conditions for loss to be experienced as traumatic. With reference to the work of Becker (1973) who identifies death as the thing we are most defended against, Kauffman highlights the extent to which the assumptive world protects individuals from the fear and anxiety resulting from the fact of our mortality. The transferential nature of the assumptive world is a theme developed by Liechty, (in Kauffman, 2003, p. 91) and Obholzer, who identifies the NHS as a primary site and focus of these most basic and existential fears referring to it as 'the keep death at bay service' (1994, p. 171).

In this way inner worlds shape the external world and collective states of mind are represented in the structure and fabric of society with social systems functioning as unconscious defences against anxiety. Understanding the transferential nature of the assumptive world as a mechanism of defence against existential anxiety supports a deeper understanding of individual and collective emotional responses to death and dying (Kauffman, 2002) and the nature of the emotional expectations placed upon our systems of care and the individuals representing them. It also makes it possible to connect with the full extent of the conflicting and painful feelings aroused in us all in response to death and dying and to recognize our collective vulnerability.

The concept of containment is particularly relevant when considering individual and collective vulnerabilities and anxieties when facing death. Containment is a theory of mental functioning that uses Klein's concept of projective identification to consider some of the earliest experiences involved in the development of the mind including the capacity for symbolic thought. Ogden describes Bion's idea of the container — contained as a theory of the way we think rather than what we think about,

> that is, how we process lived experience and what occurs psychically when we are unable to do psychological work with that experience (Ogden, 2004, p. 1354).

The earliest experiences of containment involve the mother receiving the baby's raw emotions or projections, processing them in her own mind and returning them to the baby in a more digestible state. The mother's attentive state is referred to as 'reverie' and requires emotional availability and sensitive attunement to the baby. Through the experience of being contained the baby takes in both the communication and the feeling of being understood. Containment has been recognized as essential to the processing of painful emotional experiences at any age particularly those that are too unbearable to be thought about.

> It refers to psychic processes through which painful experiences can be converted into reflective understanding rather than function as propellants for primitive defensive processes as described by Klein (1946) (Krantz, 2015, p. 59).

Defences in action

> Go, go, go, said the bird: human kind
>
> Cannot bear very much reality.
>
> (T. S. Eliot, 1974, p.190)

Thinking about the impact of close contact with end of life and death from psycho-analytic and psychoanalytically informed perspectives makes it possible to understand that we are all vulnerable to anxiety when faced with the possibility and reality of dying. Whilst a complex range of factors, including innate characteristics, life experiences, and the availability of close and supportive relationships, will determine individual vulnerabilities, the inevitable outcome of each human life remains. If, as Becker suggests, the denial of death is one of the deepest motivations of the human species, then it is likely that we defend ourselves constantly against the truth of our mortality, employing an almost unquantifiable range of strategies, determined by the nature of the defenses required to achieve sufficient psychic protection. Indeed Bion's description of 'nameless dread' (1962, p. 96) has been connected to the fear of annihilation and gives some sense of the extent of the anxiety that may be evoked.

Defences appear in many forms from the obvious to the subtle and with a range of consequences — some easily identified, others less so. In whatever way they emerge they inevitably influence and shape both the way that we behave and the way that we communicate with one another. Professional, organizational and personal defences can all be identified in situations involving close contact with death and mortality. Speck in Obholzer (1994) refers to a number of defences that might be employed to protect against the emotional impact of such work including; rationalization, intellectualization, bluntness, adopting a task centred- approach and avoidance. He also recognizes the potentially defensive nature of aggressive treatments including invasive surgery, a theme that has been taken up more recently by Gawande (2014), who writes both as a doctor and the son of a dying parent, about the limitations of modern medicine.

In addition to the defences referred to earlier Menzies Lyth's classic study of nursing in a London hospital went on to consider the role of the organization in dealing with anxiety and found that the social systems that had evolved over time within the hospital in the form of hierarchies, rules, procedures, rotas and task lists, acted as supports for these defensive techniques and mechanisms.

The following examples are drawn from the author's lived experience to illustrate some of the ideas discussed above. They represent a range of defences in action and include personal, professional, and organizational responses to end of life situations.

Having watched my father die from an aggressive cancer when my husband became ill my mind simply refused to accept the possibility that this was going to happen again. The disease I selected as an alternative was deeply unpleasant but retained the possibility of recovery. I think now that I must have been in such a state of denial that I managed to convince the consultant that this was the most likely diagnosis. On reflection I now wonder if he allowed me to believe what I needed to at the time knowing that a more accurate diagnosis was only a question of time.

From a professional perspective I recall the evening my husband had just been told that he had advanced cancer. As I arrived on the ward staff watched us from a distance looking awkward and uncomfortable whilst he told me the news himself. No one approached us not even to see if we needed anything and later that evening, the only nurse who seemed to be on duty, a young student nurse who clearly felt our pain, but lacked the experience and skills to find an appropriate response, attempted to comfort us by saying, 'Well, things can only get better.'

A few days later a Consultant Oncologist suggested a last minute intervention involving a biopsy to confirm the source of the primary tumor and we found ourselves caught in the complex territory Gawande (2014) describes so well:

> So everyone struggles with this uncertainty — with how and when, to accept that the battle is lost (Gawande, 2014, p. 157).

I have no doubt that this particular oncologist felt there was some hope and that failure to pursue this option might be interpreted as negligent. For my husband, approaching his fiftieth birthday and the father of two dependent children, the offer of hope was irresistible. The fact that the palliative care specialist at the hospice indicated that she was not hopeful but that it was up to us, suggested the procedure represented a need to do 'something'. Unable to resist at the time I had some sense of this being a way of defending himself (and us) with his potential power and even omnipotence. I now feel that perhaps we were all left with little choice but to pursue this course of action. Either way the intervention was completed three days before he died and took up a significant amount of the precious time he had remaining.

Returning to the concept of social systems as defences against anxiety I offer the example of my mother who waited for a bed in a nursing home for far longer than she should have done, this not helped by knowing that many others wait for as long, if not longer. After the 'DNR' conversation where it became apparent that without intervention my mother would most likely die on the hospital ward I asked that a referral be made to the hospice. When the hospice confirmed that a bed was available for her on a particular day the response of the system was that it would not be possible to arrange transport at such short notice and she would have to wait, possibly for forty-eight hours.

At the time this seemed to represent a complete failure of imagination or initiative and I feel almost ashamed that in drawing on my professional knowledge and experience I was able to make an arrangement that allowed her to be moved and admitted to the hospice. Before this could happen I had to agree to accept full responsibility for her during the journey, absolving the hospital of responsibility for an extremely sick and dying patient.

These are examples of some of the experiences that occur on a daily basis as individuals attempt to negotiate a way through the systems of care representing society's response to serious illness, vulnerability, dying and end of life. I hear the themes repeated in individual stories when I reveal the subject of my thesis, find them in the detail of the evidence given by patients and relatives to the inquiry that resulted in The Francis Report (2013) and most recently read about them in the latest report from the Health Ombudsman (2015). Being on the receiving end of defensive responses at times of great vulnerability and need is isolating, disorientating and demoralizing. The initial impact is immediate but the consequences of being so misunderstood and uncontained are felt over time and often with lasting effect.

It would appear that many of the complaints made about the quality of the care provided for ageing, vulnerable people including those at the end of life such as my own parents and husband, represent missiles formed from uncontained and unbearable projections. Certainly in each of the living with dying/end of life situations I have found myself in, I can recognize that at times I, and significant others, were functioning in a paranoid schizoid state of mind and more than a little psychotic at least temporarily. In serious need of professionals and systems with the capacity to contain our fear and pain we found ourselves avoided, referred on and overlooked.

Dartington (2010) hypothesizes that services around vulnerable people are influenced by two states of mind, the heroic with paranoid schizoid characteristics and the stoical with depressive position characteristics. Health care is more closely associated with the paranoid schizoid, heroic position and social care with the more depressive, stoical state of mind with a split enacted between them. In contrast my experience of hospice care suggests the possibility that individuals and organizations have the potential to move beyond the defences of the paranoid schizoid and depressive positions.

Of particular interest is Symington's identification of a third tragic position that accepts 'la condition humaine' (Symington, 1986, p. 276). Taking up the idea Lawrence (2000) suggests that whilst depressive position defences may appear more benign than those representing the paranoid schizoid position, it is only from the tragic position that we are fully able to acknowledge our mortality (Lawrence, 2000, p. 212). The concept of a third position makes it possible to understand something of what might be required for individuals and organisations to offer end of life care that is accepting of death, sensitive to the holistic needs of the dying person and those around them, and hopeful about what might be achieved in the time that remains. Exploring the idea of a third position, its existence and the conditions that might support and sustain it in different care settings including homely environments is one aspect of the author's research.

Shaping the future

The emotional terrain of end of life care is complex and dynamic. The constant interplay between conscious and unconscious states of mind, psychic positions, and their associated defences mobilized in various forms to protect against the fear, pain and anxiety stirred up by close proximity to death and dying is inevitable. The author's personal journey represents something of the variable quality of end of life care and includes examples of times when fear and anxiety were uncontained or projected back as well as times when the contained and containing presence of just one individual made the end of life meaningful and bearable. It reveals the deeply personal impact of the primary task of caring for those at the end of life on the individuals representing our systems of care.

Whilst concerns about the quality of end of life care have gathered momentum in recent years it would seem there is correspondingly little evidence to suggest that attention has been given to the emotional impact of caring for patients at the end of life. Existing systems of care are increasingly organised around complex and competing sets of priorities and within the NHS the history of attending to the emotional needs of those caring directly for patients is patchy and inconsistent. Speaking about the sustainability of informal systems of coping in nursing Langstaff and Tutton note that:

> Although our understanding of emotional labour in nursing has increased, the underpinning theoretical framework of anxiety has not been assumed into nursing developments (Tutton and Langstaff, 2015, p. 122).

It would seem that beyond the world of hospice and specialist palliative care, opportunities for the kind of containment Bion identified as essential to the capacity for reflective thinking in the presence of painful emotional experiences, are not readily available. The consequences of this lack means that even when organizations and professionals are trying hard to get it right by following standards, guidelines, and recommendations, the impact of death denying defences go unnoticed, and unremarked. Shaping a future that can support and sustain the provision of compassionate care depends upon an engagement with the unconscious aspects of human nature including ambivalence and hatred that impact on individual and organizational responses to vulnerability and mortality. The findings of Menzies Lyth are as relevant as ever. Finding the structure of the nursing system defective as a means of handling anxiety and as a method of organizing its tasks she makes the proposition that,

> The success and viability of a social institution are intimately connected with the techniques it uses to contain anxiety (Menzies, 1960, p. 118).

An understanding of the containing functions of health and social care organizations is essential for those tasked with the integrated care agenda. If these aspects of the work can be acknowledged the emphasis can be placed on systems and structures that reduce and modify anxiety instead of evading it in more primitive and pathological ways (Menzies, 1960). At the same time a willingness to transcend traditional boundaries and hierarchies will create opportunities for those more familiar with the experience of death and dying, who hold, and can support others to hold the tragic position, to contribute in innovative ways to the end of life care agenda. A focus on emotional maturity and the capacity to learn from the experience of working closely with those at end of life will support appropriate appointments and shape services that can engage fully with all aspects of end of life care.

Creating posts and specific roles where the primary task is to recognize, respond to, and regulate the emotional states of mind of all involved, offering comfort and support as and when necessary, might seem unusual but may be necessary if individuals and systems are to increase their capacity for emotionally engaged and compassionate care. The emotional capacity to be present at the end of life without resorting to unhelpful paranoid schizoid or depressive defences will make it more likely that the end of life is recognized and can be discussed appropriately.

Essential to the process will be individuals who are familiar with death, accepting of mortality (the tragic position), and who have the emotional and mental capacity to use self effectively in relationships with others. In recent years palliative care social workers have contributed to the skills and development of health and social care workers (Skills for Care, 2014) and representatives of the Association of Palliative Care Social Workers have highlighted the significant contribution that palliative care social work can make to the wider provision of end of life care (Community Care, 2008, 2014). Intimately connected with relationship based social work practice through the shared theoretical roots described earlier, the current Chair of the APCSW, Ann Cullen, describes it as 'a model of social work that's very much in keeping with the direction in which people want the profession to develop' (2014).

Placing such practice at the heart of end of life care has the potential to shift the emphasis from the bureaucratised models of service delivery and management of services that have developed throughout health and social care in recent years. Indeed Trevith-ick's discussion of the need to humanise management is perhaps as relevant to end of life care as it is to child-care social work (2014). Relationship based practice acknowledges the significance of the conscious and unconscious dimensions of human behaviour and the importance of psychosocial approaches to practice.

Relationship based approaches have a long and established history within the social work profession as does the concept of reflective practice and the conditions that sup-port it, (Ruch 2007). Social work practitioners have extensive experience of working in partnership with vulnerable people, agencies and communities and communicating about difficult and emotionally painful subjects. There is much evidence (Small, 2001; Beresford *et al.*, 2007, 2008) to suggest that the combined contribution that palliative care and relationship based social work practice can make to appropriate end of life care, is significant and worthy of further development

At the same time early findings from the author's own psychosocial doctoral re-search (Clarke and Hoggett, 2009) suggest that the move to ensure more people can end their lives in their usual place of care has identified areas of expertise and contain-ment that have been at least to some extent previously overlooked and undervalued. Interviewing care workers in non specialist settings about their experiences of end of life care has made me aware of places where sitting with the dying has become part of the culture of the home and emotional responses accepted and supported. Some of those interviewed have described the ways they have found to make the end of life a meaningful experience, demonstrating sensitive attunement to the individual con-cerned and creating rituals that reflect a person's life and represent something of the caring relationship. Indeed some of the accounts of care given at end of life have come very close to Bion's description of reverie and suggest that there is much to learn from these close encounters with the end of life.

For example the difference that a thoughtful care team made to the state of mind of a resident with dementia reaching the end of her life is difficult to quantify but never-theless significant. Her preference for sleeping on the floor was understood, accepted and honoured. Placing her mattress on the floor made up with familiar bedding created an environment that she experienced as comforting and containing.

Conclusion

Moving beyond our existing relationship with ageing, death, and dying, established over time and determined by a range of complex factors that evidence the extent of our need to deny death, has the potential to transform our society. Finding ways to engage with the emotional challenges involved will be essential to the process. The psychoanalytic perspectives offered provide some explanation of why we might be struggling to accommodate death culturally, organizationally, professionally and personally and why we need receptacles (Cooper and Lousada, 2005, p. 177) in the form of containing relationships and social systems to support us all as we try to become more familiar with the idea and fact of our mortality.

For those closely involved with end of life care, being able to remain emotionally available in the moments when patients and their families are facing the accumulated losses of end of life requires a particular kind of knowledge and experience. It requires knowledge and understanding of the complexities and ambiguities of human relationships including the defences that we all employ throughout our lives to keep ourselves safe. It also requires an awareness of, and sensitivity to, what might be stirred up in those working closely with vulnerable and dying people and to create environments and structures with the capacity to respond accordingly.

According to Holman *et al.* (2006) it is the feelings and associated psychological defences attached to the hidden and less conscious aspects of the emotional demands of care that are the key to supporting care staff in developing their capacity for caring for those at the end of life. They make a strong case for the use of emotionally containing, psychoanalytically informed, methods including supervision and reflective groups to explore hidden aspects of the caring experience in developing this capacity (Holman *et al.*, 2006). It is an approach that is relevant and applicable to many aspects of end of life care as demonstrated by Jones who acknowledges the practical value of Bion's theory of containment when applied to the role of the Macmillan nurse (Bion, 1970). Required to contain their patients' strong and unrefined emotions, they in turn require containing experiences in order to process their thoughts, feelings and impressions (Jones, 1999, p. 1302).

Psychoanalytic knowledge of group and institutional dynamics is particularly relevant when considering the need to create the kind of teams and working environments that can contain and process not only conscious and openly expressed emotions and anxiety, but also the primitive and unconscious ones we know will be aroused by the nature of end of life care. Whether or not funding and attention is directed towards the conditions required to support and develop these capabilities will determine how much progress can be made and the quality of care provided. Perhaps most significantly it will come to define the very nature of our society.

Disclosure statement

No potential conflict of interest was reported by the author.

References

Age UK. (2014) *Care in Crisis*. Available from: www.ageuk.org.uk

Aries, P. (1982) *The Hour of our Death*, Vintage Books, New York, NY.

Becker, E. (1973) *The Denial of Death*, The Free Press, New York, NY.

Beresford, P., Croft, S. & Adshead, L. (2007) *Palliative Care, Social Work and Service Users: Making Life Possible*, Jessica Kingsley, London and Philadelphia.

Beresford, P., Croft, S. & Adshead, L. (2008) '"We don't see her as a social worker". A service user case study of the importance of the social worker's relationship and humanity', *British Journal of Social Work*, vol. 38, no. 7, pp. 1388–1407.

Bion, W. R. (1970) *Attention and Interpretation: A Scientific Approach to Insight in Psychoanalysis and Groups*, Tavistock Publications Limited, London and New York.

Bower, M. (2003) 'Broken and twisted', *Journal of Social Work Practice*, vol. 17, no. 2, pp. 143–151.

Bowlby, J. (1969) *Attachment and Loss*, vol. 1, Hogarth Press, London.

Bowlby, J. (1973) *Attachment and Loss*, vol. 2, Hogarth Press, London.

Bowlby, J. (1980) *Attachment and Loss*, vol. 3, Hogarth Press, London.

Budd, S. & Rusbridger, R. (2005) 'Basic Concepts'. in *Introducing Psychoanalysis: Essential Themes and Topics*, eds S. Budd & R. Rusbridger, Routledge, London.

Clarke, S. & Hoggett, P. (2009) *Researching Beneath The Surface: Psycho-social Research Methods in Practice*, Karnac, London.

Community Care. (9 Oct 2008) *End of Life*, pp. 30–31. Available from: www.communitycare.co.uk

Community Care. (18 Feb 2014) *Adults, End of Life Care*. Available from: www.communitycare.co.uk

Cooper, A. & Lousada, J. (2005) *Borderline Welfare: Feeling and Fear of Feeling in Modern Welfare*, Karnac, London.

Dartington, T. (2010) *Managing Vulnerability: The Underlying Dynamics Of Systems Of Care*, Karnac, London.

Department of Health Online. (2008) *End of Life Care Strategy*. Available from: www.dh.gov.uk/publications

Dying Well Community Charter. (2014) Available from: www.ncpc.org.uk, www.dyingmatters.org

Eliot, T. S. (1974) *Collected Poems, 1909–1962*, Faber, London.

Francis, R. (2013) *The Mid Staffordshire NHS Foundation Trust Public Inquiry: Public Inquiry Chaired by Robert Francis QC*, HMSO, London.

Freud, S. (1912) 'The Dynamics of Transference', in *The Standard Edition Of The Complete Psychological Works*, vol. X11 (1911–1913), London: Hogarth Press Limited, 1958, pp. 97–108.

Freud, S. (1920) *A General Introduction to Psychoanalysis*, Horace Liverlight, New York.

Gawande, A. (2014) *Being Mortal: Illness, Medicine, and What Matters in the End*, Profile Books, London.

Holloway, M. (2007) *Negotiating Death*, The Policy Press, Bristol.

Holman, C., Meyer, J. & Davenhill, R. (2006) 'Psychoanalytically informed research in an NHS continuing care unit for older people: exploring and developing staff's work with complex loss and grief', *Journal of Social Work Practice*, vol. 20, no. 3, pp. 315–328.

Jones, A. (1999) '"A heavy and blessed experience": a psychoanalytic study of community Macmillan nurses and their roles in serious illness and palliative care', *Journal of Advanced Nursing*, vol. 30, no. 6, pp. 1297–1303.

Kauffman, J. ed., (2002) *Loss Of The Assumptive World: A Theory Of Traumatic Loss*, Routledge, New York, NY.

Klein, M. (1946). 'Notes on some schizoid mechanisms', in *Writings, : Envy and Gratitude and Other Works,* vol. 3, pp. 1–24. London: Hogarth Press, 1975: reprinted London: Karnac, 1993.

Klein, M. (1975) *Envy and Gratitude and Other Works 1946–1963*, eds R. Khan & M. Masud, The Hogarth Press and Institute of Psychoanalysis, London.

Krantz, J. (2015) 'Social defences in the information age', in *Social Defences Against Anxiety: Explorations in a Paradigm*, vol. 3, eds D. Armstrong & M. Rustin, Karnac, London.

Kubler-Ross, E. (1969) *On Death and Dying*, Tavistock, London.

Lawrence, G. (2000) *Tongued with Fire: Groups in Experience*, Karnac, London.

Leadership Alliance for the Care of Dying People. (2014) *One Chance to Get it Right: Improving People's Experience of Care in the Last Few Days and Hours of Life*. Available from: www.gov.uk/publications

Menzies, I. E. P. (1960) 'A case-study in the functioning of social systems as a defence against anxiety: a report on a study of the nursing service of a general hospital', *Human Relations*, vol. 13, no. 2, pp. 95–121.

Murray-Parkes, C. (1998) *Bereavement: Studies of Grief in Adult Life*, 3rd ed, Tavistock Publications, London.

National Council for Palliative Care. (2014) *The End of Life Care Strategy: New Ambitions*. Available from: www.ncpc.org.uk

Nice. (2011/2013) *QS13 End of Life Care for Adults*. Available from: www.publications.nice.org.uk

Ogden, T. H. (2004) 'On Holding and Containing, Being and Dreaming', *International Journal of Psychoanalysis*, vol. 85, no. 6, pp. 1349–1364.

Parliamentary and Health Service Ombudsman. (2015) *Dying Without Dignity: Investigations by the Parliamentary and Health Service Ombudsman into complaints about end of life care*. Available from: www.ombudsman.org.uk

Ruch, G. (2007) 'Reflective practice in contemporary child-care social work: the role of containment', *British Journal of Social Work*, vol. 37, no. 4, pp. 659–680.

Saunders, C. ed. (1990) *Hospice and Palliative Care: An Interdisciplinary Approach*, Edward Arnold, London.

Sheldon, F. (1997) *Psychosocial Palliative Care: Good Practice in the Care of the Dying and Bereaved*, Stanley Thorne Publishers Ltd, Surrey.

Skills for Care. (2014) *Evaluation of Yorkshire and the Humber End of Life Care Development Programme for Care Homes*, Final Report, 2014. Available from: www.skillsforcare.org.uk

Small, N. (2001) 'Social Work and Palliative Care', *British Journal of Social Work*, vol. 31, pp. 961–971.

Speck, P. (1994) in *The Unconscious at Work: Individual and Organizational Stress in the Human Services*, ed A. Obholzer, Routledge: London, pp. 94–100.

Symington, N. (1986) *The Analytic Experience: Lectures from the Tavistock*, Free Association Books, London.

Trevithick, P. (2014) 'Humanising managerialism: Reclaiming emotional reasoning, intuition, the relationship, and knowledge and skills in social work', *Journal of Social Work Practice*, vol. 3, no. 6, pp. 287–311.

Tutton, L. & Langstaff, D. (2015) 'Reflections on Isabel Menzies Lyth in the light of developments in nursing care', in *Social Defences Against Anxiety: Explorations in a Paradigm*, eds D. Armstrong & M. Rustin, Karnac, London, pp. 111–123.

Walter, T. (1994) *The Revival of Death*, Routledge, London.

Worden, W. (1991) *Grief and Grief Therapy: A Handbook for the Mental Health Practitioner*, Routledge, Oxford.

Sue Taplin

'LIVING TO TELL THE TALE' — NARRATIVES OF SURVIVING CANCER AND THE SOCIAL WORK RESPONSE

This article draws on themes derived from research conducted as part of my doctoral study with eighteen individuals who were living with cancer, in which they were invited to explore the ways in which they experienced the world around them, how it had affected their sense of self and their relationships with others and whether and in what ways it had given them a different perspective on the present and the future. This research developed from my practice as a Social Worker in Palliative Care, during which time I became fascinated by the different reactions and responses which individual people displayed to a diagnosis of life-threatening illness, and how these changed during the trajectory of the illness, and specifically, in people living with a diagnosis of cancer, which did not always result in death. Drawing on interviews with cancer 'survivors', the concepts of biographical disruption, liminality and survivorship are explored as a means of understanding the reality of living with cancer. Finally there is a discussion of the implications of the research for contemporary social work practice.

The special case of cancer

For many years, and significantly even in contemporary society, a cancer diagnosis has been seen by many as a 'death warrant'. Cancer has occupied such an invidious place in the public imagination that the association between cancer and death is now well entrenched in popular myth (McNamara, 2001, p. 28). Kellehear (1990, p. 65) suggested that, if you are diagnosed with cancer, both 'popular and professional views … define you as dying'.

According to McNamara (2001), it is no wonder that misinformation and fear about cancer takes root in contemporary western societies, as there are a multiplicity of messages about the disease which inevitably create uncertainty. These messages are presented in both professional and lay discourse. We are told of the hope that exists in new cures and therapies and of the drawn-out deaths of those who have 'lost the battle' against the 'dreaded' disease. 'Messages of hope and despair combine, fuelling a cultural terror and exposing our inherent fragility, our fear of death' (McNamara, 2001, p. 28).

The newly diagnosed cancer patient is debilitated not only by the *symptoms* of the disease, but also by the *symbols* of the disease. Cancer is associated with pollution, with uncontrollable and overwhelming growth, and with evil. ... It is not that we are unsympathetic to the cancer sufferer, it is that cancer has a life beyond the particular disease (McNamara, 2001, p. 29).

McNamara (2001, p. 31) suggests that one of the reasons why cancer is so feared is the fact that its causation is still not established. Despite numerous clinical studies which have indicated connections between, for example, chronic stress and cancer and between relationship losses and cancer onset (Selye, 1986), findings which propose emotional, psychological and social factors to be significant causes of cancer can be seen as highly contentious. As such the mystery remains and cancer continues to be viewed as something which cannot be understood or tamed.

Field (1996, p. 256) suggests that cancer is associated with fear and mystery for a number of different reasons, notably, the unexpectedness and untimeliness of its appearance. Although it is not unusual for cancer sufferers to interpret their cancer as a warning to review and change their lifestyles, this understanding is usually constructed in retrospect and it is unlikely that many people expect to get cancer. Likewise, a diagnosis of cancer is often 'untimely', in that it subverts our normal expectations of longevity and as such the threat of death before the 'due' time is all the more difficult to deal with.

According to McNamara (2001, p. 33) 'whether we are fatalistic or vigilant in our monitoring of cancer risks, whether we favour reductionist biomedical explanations or psychologically based explanations like the 'typical' cancer personality, we still cannot seem to escape the association between cancer and death. They are an unfortunate pair and the myth continues despite advances in cancer control and the hope that exists in the hearts of so many cancer sufferers'.

Traditional understandings of illnesses such as cancer representing a 'death sentence' are continually challenged as contemporary healthcare confronts the frontiers of treatment and cure. However, even though death rates of once predictable terminal illnesses are falling, many people are living with the aftermath of the illness itself and/ or the treatment regimens. Chronic illness and associated morbidities, together with the ageing of populations in many industrialised countries, have the potential to change the community's demands on healthcare systems.

How, then, should we respond to the changing nature of cancer in Western society, and what theories of understanding are available to us to help us develop practice with people who are living with this disease?

The role and responsibility of social work to people living with cancer

According to Small (2001, p. 961) 'there are close links between the philosophy and practice of palliative care and that of social work' and social work has a particular contribution to make to the care of people who are living with life-threatening illness in three main respects: that this experience inevitably involves loss, and social work has always been concerned with responding to loss; that social work brings a 'whole system' approach, putting individual experience into a wider context; and that social work is concerned with helping people to ameliorate the practical impact of change. What characterises social work in the context of life-threatening illness is its ability to recognise the holistic needs of individuals and families, and how, despite recent trends towards care management in mainstream social work (Lloyd, 1997, 2002), palliative care social work has largely managed to retain its traditional casework approach, so valued by service users, as evidenced by Beresford *et al.* (2007).

In my experience as a social worker in a hospice from 1995 to 2004, the role of the social worker complemented that of the multi-disciplinary team by ensuring that a psychosocial model of care was offered to patients and families alongside the medical model, and service users were encouraged to identify and achieve self-defined goals, to fulfil their potential and to 'live', rather than simply 'survive', for as long as was possible — essentially an individualised approach to care was provided which counteracted some of the more restrictive aspects of the medical interventions which service users would often have to undergo.

However, Clausen *et al.* (2005) found that, in their study, although many patients and carers had expressed psychosocial needs, which could clearly be met by social workers, few, if any, had any social work involvement. This was partly attributed to a lack of understanding on the part of the wider team about the roles and tasks of social work, and a reluctance on the part of potential service users to request a social work assessment, fearing the social stigma associated with this. Nevertheless, Beresford *et al.*'s (2007) research determined that what palliative care service users who had received social work intervention desired from and valued about the service was the ability and willingness of the worker to 'journey' with them, providing continuity of care and acting as a guide into the unknown (Beresford *et al.*, 2007; Reith and Payne, 2009).

The challenge to social work today would seem to be for agencies, organisations and individual practitioners to recognise the changing world of cancer care and to enable social workers to reach out to those who are living with, as well as dying from, cancer, recognising that the need for psychosocial intervention and support is on-going and that the same skills that are valued by those who are dying may be equally as applicable to those who are surviving.

Exploring the experience of living with cancer — three conceptual frameworks

Through listening to the stories of individuals who are living with cancer and from my review of research studies on the experience of living with life-threatening illness, and specifically cancer, I have discerned three major concepts which may serve to enhance the practitioner's understanding of this experience. These are, as follows, biographical disruption, liminality and survivorship.

Biographical disruption and cancer

The concept of biographical disruption was introduced into the discourse by Bury in 1982 as a means both to describe people's experiences of chronic illness and as a framework to understand how people respond and adapt to such illness (Lawton, 2003;

Hubbard *et al.*, 2010) More recently, however, researchers in the field of cancer have sought to explore the potential of this concept for understanding the experience of living with cancer. Cancer has traditionally been conceptualised as an acute illness, but with the advances in earlier diagnosis and improved treatment of cancer, more people are living longer with the consequences of cancer, and thus it is a disease which may be seen increasingly to fall within the category of a chronic condition. The core condition for biographical disruption, as defined by Bury in 1982, is that it is precipitated by a disruptive event, a major disruptive experience or a critical situation. In cancer, the onset of illness can be seen to 'disrupt' people's assumptions about their bodies, themselves and the social world in which they live, and bring to the fore thoughts of pain, suffering and death, which are normally only considered to be distant or remote possibilities in life which can be ignored or are perceived as things that happen to other people. Thus, according to Cayless *et al.* (2010), while biographical disruption has not usually been applied to acute illness, it can be seen to be a useful concept for describing and explaining people's experiences of cancer, particularly within the first year.

Furthermore, I would argue that biographical disruption is a relevant concept for describing and explaining the experience of cancer for some individuals because a diagnosis of cancer can represent a threat to identity.

Like Bury, Charmaz (1994) suggests that chronic illness raises people's awareness of death and disrupts their perception of themselves, particularly if the individual considers him or herself too young to die, or defines themselves as healthy and has no personal experience of illness within which to contextualise the experience. This concept of disruption, which can be seen as an assault on the 'self', has been applied directly to the experience of cancer, for example, in studies by Exley and Letherby (2001) and Shaha and Cox (2003). Disruption of a person's biography can affect not only how people view themselves but also how they think they are viewed by other people. It can lead to social isolation and a sense of 'difference' from contemporaries (Cayless *et al.*, 2010). This again is a characteristic of the experience of living with cancer, as will become evident in the stories of my respondents.

Bury's concept of coping is also relevant here, as it refers to cognitive processes whereby individuals learn to manage their illness and 'involves maintaining a sense of value and meaning in life, in spite of symptoms and their effects' (Bury, 1991, p. 461). Examples of coping include normalisation and 'bracketing off' the impact of the illness so that the effects on identity are minimised. According to Bury (2001) there are two processes of normalisation. People may normalise in the sense of trying to keep their pre-illness lifestyle and identity intact by either maintaining as many pre-illness activities as possible and/or by disguising and minimising symptoms. Other people find ways to incorporate their illness into an altered lifestyle so that 'normal' life is reorientated around the illness, thus 'containing' it.

The analysis of the literature of biographical disruption aids our understanding of possible issues for those who are living with cancer and provides a potential framework for intervention in this still somewhat unchartered new territory. Biographically informed approaches to care complement a narrow medical focus on the body and physical symptoms and present the opportunity to broaden our understanding of illness to include social and spiritual dimensions, and as such to support individuals to manage the psychosocial consequences of their diagnosis.

Liminality

Kleinman (1988) has documented the 'apartness' of people who are seriously ill with particular clarity in his work on illness narratives. This state of 'apartness' has also been termed 'liminality' and can be seen as a territory which the survivor of serious illness enters and which persists in some form or other for the rest of the person's life. It resembles the state referred to by Frank (1995, pp. 8–13) as membership of the 'remission society'. It is a concept which derives from social anthropology and seems originally to have been used by van Gennep (1960) in his 1909 study of rites of passage. For van Gennep, rituals marked a process of 'passing through' a phase of social evolution. During a period of separation from the rest of society, the person was prepared by purification. This phase of separation was followed by a phase of transition, when the initiate had left their former state, but had not yet entered the new one. This stage was termed by van Gennep as *liminaire,* meaning 'of the threshold' (Little *et al.*, 1998).

Turner elaborates on the meaning of the term, referring to it as a state of being 'betwixt and between the normal, day to day, cultural and social states', an identifiable space in which normal societal roles and status may be relinquished or taken away.

In the context of illness, Frankenberg (1986) follows Turner in using the term to describe periods of disruption in life caused by illness, in which structure and routine are abandoned. Murphy *et al.* used the term to describe the social view of people with chronic disability as in a state which was 'cloudy and indeterminate' (p. 238). For Little *et al.* (1998), however, liminality is not seen as a phase to be passed through, but rather as an 'enduring and variable state' and as such, 'the labelling inherent in the cancer diagnosis is sufficient to induce and maintain liminality' (Little *et al.*, 1998, p. 1490). Within the context that Little *et al.* apply to liminality in relation to cancer, and based on their research with adults living with colorectal cancer, it can be experienced in two stages — the immediate phase of acute liminality (upon diagnosis) and an enduring phase of sustained liminality, which may last for the rest of the individual's life.

The moment one suspects that something is wrong is when one enters the liminality or 'crosses the threshold' of cancer. With the diagnosis of a potentially fatal illness one is 'set apart' from others who do not have the same concentration of mind on their own mortality. As mentioned earlier, Little *et al.* (1998) distinguish between two stages of liminality. The initial acute phase begins when an individual's suspicions that something is wrong are confirmed, when he or she hears the 'bad' news and experiences the existential threat.

Sustained liminality follows the acute phase at an indeterminate time, depending on a variety of physical, social and psychosocial factors, including how the individual managed the acute phase, the availability and acceptance of external support, to what extent the diagnosis represented a disruption to the biography of the individual, and the impact and outcome of the treatment. Patients in this phase begin to regain control over some aspects of their lives whilst remaining aware of their 'differentness' from others. People who have had cancer remain identified as people who have (experienced) cancer, regardless of whether they accept this identification: '... they enter, along with sufferers from chronic illness and those who have survived serious threats to life, a phase of sustained liminality, in which adaptive mechanisms are repeatedly formulated and reformulated' (Little *et al.*, 1998, p. 1493; see also Tishelman and Sachs, 1992). 'Cancer changes the sufferer's life forever, for even if that person is able to go on living, he or she lives under threat of possible recurrence of the disease' (McNamara, 2001, pp. 33–34).

An exploration of liminality is useful to this study because it provides another means of understanding the dynamic processes of accommodation and adaptation that a person living with cancer may be required to undergo. In common with biographical disruption and survivorship (below), liminality is a concept which has at its core the significance of individual experience, while at the same time offering a broad and flexible interpretive framework within which to understand that experience (Little *et al.*, 2006; Cayless *et al.*, 2010).

Survivorship

The term survivorship first appeared in the medical literature in the 1960s with reference to life after myocardial infarction (Lew, 1967). By the 1980s the concept of survivorship had begun to appear in cancer-related literature, incorporating not only the notion of *biomedical* survival but also the *psychosocial* perspective, although it was mainly limited to the experience of paediatric survivors reaching adulthood (Jaffe, 1975; Doyle, 2008). Nevertheless, according to Doyle (2008) there has been little progress in the conceptualisation of cancer survivorship, despite the significant rise in the number of cancer survivors, and the term continues to be used interchangeably with related terms, such as 'people living with/through cancer'.

Due to developments in public health policy in terms of screening and early detection, together with more effective treatments, increasing numbers of people in industrialised countries with once terminal illnesses such as cancer consider themselves (or are considered to be) 'survivors'. However, seeking a definition of 'survivor' is difficult, since there is subjectivity to this status as well as a changing professional understanding, depending on different phases of illness and treatment.

Little *et al.* recognise the ambivalent nature of the concept of survivorship, contrasting 'the inspirational literature about individual resilience with that of the difficulty of 'being' a survivor' (cited in O'Connor, 2008, p. 115), the latter of which may involve feelings of vulnerability to the ever-present possibility of recurrence and by the possible subsequent impact of this on all aspects of life. Shanfield (1980) concluded that the cancer experience was a permanent one, not just limited to the treatment phase, but characterised instead by ongoing vivid memories of the illness and recovery period, coupled with an enduring sense of one's own mortality and vulnerability (Doyle, 2008).

Little *et al.* (2000) connect the concepts of liminality and survivorship by describing the potentially life-changing nature of the cancer experience, in that 'cancer survivors pass through the space of illness but do not return to their world as it was before the illness' (Doyle, 2008, p. 503). Payne suggests that survivors 'have to simultaneously inhabit the world of the 'healthy' population and the world of the patient' (Payne, 2007, p. 430), which suggests a sense of having to exist within two communities and the need somehow to be able to cross the divide, as in the state of liminality, described above. The extent to which individuals are able to 'bridge' this gap or how far the feelings of 'otherness' dominate will affect how far they feel integrated or isolated as a cancer 'survivor'.

The reality of living with cancer

In the interviews I conducted with people living with cancer, I observed for myself how far their experience 'fits' the conceptual frameworks described above, as individuals navigated their own paths through cancer. For the purpose of this article, I have selected three of the most significant themes, namely, the role of spirituality and meaning-making, the significance of occupation, and relationships with others.

The significance of spirituality and meaning-making

What could be seen as a protective factor for a number of respondents, and which could account for their apparent acceptance of the situation, was their Christian faith. For one respondent, Fiona, a 76 year old retired pharmacist with cancer of the spine, it was the belief in an afterlife which gave her hope and reduced her fear, whereas for Margaret, of similar age, a retired nurse with cancer of the breast, who had been widowed and then remarried, it was the prayers of her local Church members.

The faith or belief system which was deemed to be supportive and helpful in managing the experience of cancer was also reported by a number of younger respondents, for example, for Brenda (a single woman in her 50s with ovarian cancer who had taken early retirement on health grounds) who recognised that support from Church members appeared to increase once she was diagnosed with an illness they could understand, rather than the mental health difficulties she also experienced. For Robert, separated, aged 57, with cancer of the blood, who had trained as a social worker and was, at the time of diagnosis, managing a social work team, faith was a personal matter; it gave him strength, as did Quakerism for Mo (a 42 year old married statistician with breast cancer) and Buddhism for Jean (a 65 year old retired youth worker/counsellor with cancer of the bladder who now lived alone). For Faye, a 2 years married mother of two young children, trained as a physiotherapist but currently not working, her Christian faith meant that she felt part of a community of believers, who she found to be supportive. Both Lisa (a single 49 year old practising social worker) and Fiona (above) had encounters with Christian medical professionals who shared their faith and were prepared to disclose it, which both respondents found helpful.

Spirituality was a common secondary theme in Foley *et al.*'s research into long-term cancer survivors, but, unlike my respondents, they found that most individuals who felt they had experienced personal growth linked this directly with spiritual growth, indicating that they had 'grown spiritually and developed a deeper appreciation or commitment to their faith' (p. 252). Halstead and Fernsler (1994, cited in Breaden, 1997, p. 983) found that in their study of 59 cancer survivors, over two-thirds of the people thought that prayer or a belief in God was a very helpful strategy in survival. However, in my study, the theme of personal growth, which characterises many of the accounts of my respondents, cannot be attributed to any particular belief or faith pattern, as it was observed in those who professed no faith as much as in those who did. Perhaps it is the ability to find meaning, to make sense of traumatic events or adverse circumstances, rather than a faith or belief in a certain religion, that makes the experience of survival more bearable (Taylor, 1995; Carter, 1993; also Frankl, 1963). However, it would be wrong to place this need to find meaning in the experience of ill health outside the realm of spirituality: indeed, meaning-seeking and meaning-taking are core components of the contemporary discourse on humanistic spirituality. According to Holloway and Moss (2010, p. 110): 'There is probably not a definition of spirituality in contemporary discourse which does not include within it the *search for meaning*'. Thompson (2010) also makes this point, observing that 'spirituality is fundamentally about meaning-making' and he links this directly to social work practice, thus emphasising the relevance of social work to addressing the needs of people living with cancer, with its emphasis on 'helping people develop more empowering meanings, understandings or 'narratives" (Thompson, 2010, p. 142, cited in Holloway and Moss, 2010, p. 7).

The significance of occupation

Work and occupation were relevant to a number of respondents of working age. The issues inherent in 'feeling different' but not wanting to be given 'preferential' treatment were highlighted as significant, as well as the difficulty of not being in control of how one is perceived by others, and how much, if anything, to disclose.

For one of the respondents, Teresa, a 56 year old married mother of two teenagers with a diagnosis of breast cancer, who was an administrator who had returned to her former workplace, there seemed to be no acknowledgement by her colleagues of the fact that she had been undergoing cancer treatment:

'Treatment finished in January and I was back at work in February, and not even on a phased return ... The first day I was back the person that did part of my work came into my office with a load of files, plonked them down on my desk and said 'thank goodness you're back, over to you!' Although Teresa appreciated not being given 'special' treatment, she felt that the fact that no acknowledgement was given to how she may be feeling was not entirely helpful.

On his return to work, Robert faced the problem of others' concern and curiosity and the issue of private information in the public sphere:

So the general story I was telling people was that ... I had a haematological issue ... I ... didn't want to give them any diagnosis and the main reasons were that firstly I was protecting myself ... and also I didn't want them looking up details about my illness ... I wasn't protecting them particularly, I didn't want them to know more than me ...

Some respondents saw their absence from work as an opportunity, when they were well enough, to leave their pre-diagnosis occupation and take up a new challenge. Dee, for example, a 56 year old woman with breast cancer, separated from her partner and with a teenage son, who had previously worked in a supermarket petrol station, decided to re-train as a beautician, thus fulfilling a long-held dream. She made the decision not to tell her new colleagues about her cancer, and the fact that she had had a mastectomy, but this was not without consequences, as she found when she had to attend a residential training course: '... I had a bedroom to myself because I didn't want to be having to get undressed in front of somebody ... but ... all the other girls wanted to know why I had got a bedroom to myself ... and I thought 'why should I keep having to explain myself?' So the general story I was telling people was that ... I had a haematological issue ... I ... didn't want to give them any diagnosis and the main reasons were that firstly I was protecting myself ... and also I didn't want them looking up details about my illness ... I wasn't protecting them particularly, I didn't want them to know more than me ...'

The significance of others — roles and identities

Of significance here is the extent to which the respondents chose to identify themselves with the 'cancer community' or to pursue their own course through the phase of illness and carry on with life as 'normal'. Some displayed the ability to move between the two worlds (that of the ill and that of the well), for example, Faye, who by turns identified with and supported a friend who was dying from cancer, but also chose to keep a part of her life separate from the experience, by not disclosing the fact of her cancer to another group of acquaintances. On one occasion, Faye refused to remove her wig even in the steamy environment of the school swimming gala as it would then 'betray' her by disclosing her identity as a person with cancer; the uncomfortable effects of the action were outweighed in Faye's mind by the fact that by doing this she was accepted as 'normal' by the other parents and could preserve her pre-cancer identity.

Some respondents were desirous not to disclose their diagnosis: Dean, a 38 year old married father of young children, living with a brain tumour and working (when health permitted) as a manager in a factory, actively sought to protect his children from a knowledge of his diagnosis, and Robert attempted to conceal his health problems from his work colleagues. 'For many respondents the emotional work they were involved with was similar to Goffman's concept of covering, whereby individuals who are both aware of their stigma and prepared to accept it '... may nonetheless make a great effort to keep the stigma from looming large" (Goffman, 1990, p. 125). Thus individuals appeared to want to detract attention from their own status, not only to maintain the illusion of 'normality' but also to reaffirm their own more valued identities of parent or manager. Kagawa-Singer also discovered this attitude in her research with people living with cancer, quoting one respondent as saying: 'I am really very healthy, I just have this problem, but I am still me' (1993, p. 295).

Susie, a 70 year old with breast cancer, with one married daughter and now living alone, also recognised that she needed to be careful when making new friendships with other people who had cancer, as she knew that the friendship was likely to be threatened by time. Young *et al.* (1999) examined friendships among women who had been diagnosed with cancer and their friends, and concluded that this is a complex area of negotiation and re-negotiation, where some women deliberately made new friends — 'friends for death, so to speak' (Young *et al.*, 1999, p. 269) — with the possibility of 'survivor guilt' when death came sooner for one than the other. The uncertainty around managing friendships for my respondents is linked by Young *et al.* (1998) to the concept of liminality, in that the sense of living 'in limbo' means that the normal 'rules' governing friendships and other social processes do not apply and new ones must continually be negotiated.

The survivorship journey

The experience of survivorship being compared metaphorically to a 'journey' is common in many cancer narratives (Breaden, 1997, p. 982). However, Breaden, in common with the majority of respondents in my study, found that this journey was

anything but linear. It was a journey that had unlit alley ways and dead end streets... There was no path *to* survival as this would imply an end to the journey. Each of the

... [respondents] were already surviving and would continue to do so for as long as each one of them lived. They did not have to wait for a specified end-point to be considered a survivor. (ibid, 1997, p. 982)

For some, there is a very real sense of being given a 'second chance', a form of re-incarnation, of experiencing life in a new way, of being a 'nicer' person, more in tune with oneself and less willing to succumb to the stresses and demands of everyday life and there is the opportunity to 'live' as opposed to merely exist or survive. Some respondents deliberately and consciously created a new life for themselves, in terms of changing career or adopting a healthier lifestyle, with the possibility of forming new relationships with their re-constructed identities. Others continued to live in much the same manner as before, but with a renewed sense of purpose and meaning. Still others, however, did not conform to any typology, and did not report any significant changes brought about by their experience. Thus, for some, the theory that the experience of cancer can create biographical disruption holds true, whereas others (a minority) may experience biographical flow or continuity, albeit with a temporary interruption.

It must be noted that this group of people, the respondents in my study, were relatively long-term 'survivors' and thus their recollections must be seen in that light — the length of time that had passed since their initial diagnosis of cancer had given them the opportunity to be thoughtful, reflective and articulate about the experience. These individuals had confronted their own mortality and had not been defeated, but they did not come through the experience unscathed, and there was for some the nagging fear that the cancer may return, which put some at least in a state of liminality. Those who viewed their experience of cancer as overwhelmingly positive and life-changing demonstrated aspects of the 'survivorship' status, but chose not to identify themselves with the term, preferring instead (if they wish to be defined at all) as saying that they were 'living with and beyond cancer'.

It is significant to note that many respondents recognised that the positive lifestyle changes they had made since the cancer were not necessarily long-lasting, for example, the restricted diet they had assumed or the way of 'living in the present' and not thinking or worrying about the future. However, a number of respondents were able to make statements such as: 'I actually think it was one of the best things that could have happened to me' and 'cancer is an emotional journey but has helped me to live my life in a more honest way ... cancer has been one of the most positive things that has ever happened to me. It's been an incredible journey and has enriched my life in ways I would never have thought possible'.

For many of the respondents, the sense of joy at still being alive seems to have outweighed other difficulties, for example, managing new relationships or the pain of treatment and subsequent after-effects, and this is borne out by Dee's exclamation part way through her interview: 'but still I am alive!' Dee had previously internalised society's view of cancer as a death sentence (Halstead and Fernsler, 1994, p. 94) but had revised her opinion in the light of her own and others' continued existence. The sense of reincarnation, of being spared to have a second chance at life is corroborated in Sekse *et al.*'s research with women five years after having been treated for gynaecological cancer: 'Gratitude for being alive was a strong issue, despite side effects and other problems following cancer treatment. The women felt they had been granted life as a gift for the second time' (Sekse *et al.*, 2010, p. 291). However, according to Breaden (1997, p. 982) the expression of feeling 'lucky to be alive', which she also found as a recurring theme in her study of cancer survivors, could also become a burden to those who had survived cancer, as they may feel unable to express feelings of ambivalence and fear lest they be somehow labelled as ungrateful or demanding.

The feeling of needing to live in the present and of reduced anxiety over trivial matters was also a common theme in my interviews. Again, Sekse *et al.* found that many of their respondents' basic values had changed as a result of their cancer experience: 'Joy for life itself and being present in their lives became important, followed by a greater stability of mood, a more positive approach to life and the ability to distinguish more clearly between important and less important matters' (Sekse *et al.*, 2010, p. 291). Nevertheless the uncertainty associated with cancer survival would seem to be ever-present, in the accounts of my respondents and also those in other research studies — as Vachon has so powerfully described it, the sense of "Waiting for the other shoe to drop' — the fear of cancer returning' (Vachon, 2001, p. 281, cited in Doyle and Kelly, 2005, p. 149).

Messages from research — implications for contemporary practice

In conclusion, then, what does this research have to say to contemporary health and social care practitioners in general, and to social workers in particular, in relation to people who are living with cancer as a long-term condition?

Cancer is clearly a condition that crosses the health and social care divide, and thus the (after) care of those who have experienced cancer in the past and are now living with its long-term effects may be significantly threatened by current austerity measures and cutbacks. According to Ham *et al.* 2012, vii (cited in Lymbery and Postle, 2015, p. 153) 'Unprecedented funding pressures affecting health and social care mean that incremental changes to current models of care will not be sufficient to address … [the] challenges. A much bolder approach is needed, involving a major shift in where care is delivered and how patients and service users relate to health and social care professionals'. It could be argued that the 2014 Care Act could offer a glimmer of hope to people living with and beyond cancer, in that the new general duty to promote well-being would seem to decree that any commissioning activity must take account of both the positive and negative impacts of a history of life-threatening illness on an individual's current sense of wellbeing; it could be argued that preserving well-being is an intrinsic part of living 'as well as one can' with cancer, and that any future assessment of a person who has experienced cancer must take account of the possible long-term effects of the illness, both physical and emotional.

My intention is that this article has highlighted the fact that the experience of cancer is poorly understood in contemporary UK society and that the journey from diagnosis to 'survivorship' may be characterised by uncertainty and fear, but that it can also be a life-changing experience for those concerned, incorporating both positive and negative aspects. There are many lessons to be learned, for example, about how the diagnosis is communicated and what support is appropriate to people who are 'living with and beyond cancer' — but essentially there needs to be a recognition that this is an individual experience that needs to be managed with sensitivity. According to Grenier

(2006, p. 310) '[p]ractitioners' increasing sense of how an event of impairment, illness or crisis is experienced, and the perception of crossing the threshold into frailty, may help them make more appropriate interventions.' Good practice in this field must be based on listening to the stories of individual people who have survived cancer and who have (literally) 'lived to tell the tale'. Social workers, whose interventions are based on psychosocial holistic care, would seem to be well-placed to provide effective and appropriate support to people who have survived cancer, to help them as individuals to make sense of living in a state of liminality, and to recognise the complexities of a disrupted biography, both for the person with cancer and for their families and friends.

Disclosure statement

No potential conflict of interest was reported by the author.

References

Beresford, P, Adshead, L & Croft, S (2007) Palliative Care, Social Work and Service Users — Making Life Possible, Jessica Kingsley, London.

Breaden, K. (1997) 'Cancer and beyond: the question of survivorship', *Journal of Advanced Nursing*, vol. 26, pp. 978–984.

Bury, M. (1982) 'Chronic illness as biographical disruption', *Sociology of Health and Illness*, vol. 4, pp. 167–182.

Bury, M. (1991) 'The sociology of chronic illness: a review of research and prospects', *Sociology of Health and Illness*, vol. 13, pp. 451–468.

Bury, M. (2001) 'Illness narratives: fact or fiction?', *Sociology of Health and Illness*, vol. 23, pp. 263–285.

Carter, B. J. (1993) 'Long-term survivors of breast cancer', *Cancer Nursing*, vol. 16, pp. 354–361.

Cayless, S., Forbat, L., Illingworth, N., Hubbard, G. & Kearney, N. (2010) 'Men with prostate cancer over the first year of illness: their experiences as biographical disruption', *Supportive Care in Cancer*, vol. 18, no. 1, pp. 11–19.

Charmaz, K. (1994) 'Identity dilemmas of chronically ill men', *The Sociological Quarterly*, vol. 35, pp. 269–288.

Clausen, H., Kendall, M., Murray, S., Worth, A. Boyd, K. & Benton, F. (2005) 'Would palliative care patients benefit from social workers' retaining the traditional 'casework' role rather than working as care managers? A prospective serial qualitative interview study', *British Journal of Social Work*, vol. 35, no. 2, pp. 277–285.

Doyle, N. & Kelly, D. (2005) "So what happens now?', *Clinical Effectiveness in Nursing*, vol. 9, pp. 147–153.

Doyle, N. (2008) 'Cancer survivorship: evolutionary concept analysis', *Journal of Advanced Nursing*, vol. 62, no. 4, pp. 499–509.

Exley, C. & Letherby, G. (2001) 'Managing a disrupted lifecourse: issues of identity and emotion work', *Health*, vol. 5, pp. 112–132.

Field, D. (1996) 'Awareness and modern dying', *Mortality*, vol. 1, pp. 255–265.

Frank, A. W. (1995) *The Wounded Storyteller: Body, Illness and Ethics*, University of Chicago, Chicago, IL.

Frankenberg, R. (1986) "Sickness as cultural performance: drama, trajectory and pilgrimage: root metaphors and the making social of disease', *International Journal of Health Services*, vol. 16, no. 4, pp. 603–626.

Frankl, V. (1963) *Man's search for meaning : an introduction to logotherapy*, Pocket Books, New York, NY.

van Gennep, A. (1960) *The Rites of Passage*, Chicago, IL, University of Chicago Press.

Goffman, E. (1990) *The Presentation of Self in Everyday Life*, Penguin, London.

Grenier, A. (2006) 'The distinction between being and feeling frail: exploring emotional experiences in health and social care', *Journal of Social Work Practice*, vol. 20, no. 3, pp. 299–313.

Halstead, M. T. & Fernsler, J. I. (1994) 'Coping strategies of long-term cancer survivors', *Cancer Nursing*, vol. 17, no. 2, pp. 94–100.

Ham, C., Dixon, A. & Brooke, B. (2012) *Transforming the Delivery of Health and Social Care - The case for fundamental change*, The Kings Fund, London.

Holloway, M. & Moss, B. (2010) *Spirituality and Social Work*, Palgrave Macmillan, Basingstoke.

Hubbard, G., Kidd, I. & Kearney, N. (2010) 'Disrupted lives and threats to identity: the experiences of people with colorectal cancer within the first year of diagnosis', *Health*, vol. 14, no. 2, pp. 131–146.

Kagawa-Singer, M. (1993) 'Redefining health: living with cancer', *Social Science and Medicine*, vol. 37, no. 3, pp. 295–304.

Kellehear, A. (1990) *Dying of Cancer: the Final Year of Life*, Harwood, London.

Kleinman, A. (1988) *The Illness Narratives: Suffering. Healing and The Human Condition*: Basic Books, New York, NY.

Lawton, J. (2003) 'Lay experiences of health and illness: past research and future agendas', *Sociology of Health and Illness*, vol. 25, pp. 23–40.

Lew, E.A. (1967) 'Survivorship after myocardial infarction', *American Journal of Public Health*, vol. 57, no. 1, pp. 118–127.

Little, M., Jordens, C.F., Paul, K., Montgomery, K. & Philipson, B. (1998) 'Liminality: a major category in the experience of cancer illness', *Social Science and Medicine*, vol. 47, no. 10, pp. 1485–1494.

Little, M., Sayers, E.J., Paul, K. & Jordens, F. (2000) 'On Surviving Cancer', *Journal of the Royal Society of Medicine*, vol. 93, no. 10, pp. 501–503.

Lloyd, M. (1997) "Dying and Bereavement', Spirituality and Social Work in a mixed economy of welfare', *British Journal of Social Work*, vol. 27, no. 2, pp. 175–190.

Lloyd, M. (2002) 'A framework for working with loss', in *Loss and Grief : A Guide for Human Services Practitioners*, ed N. Thompson, Palgrave, London, 208–220.

Lymbery, M. & Postle, K. (2015) *Social Work and the Transformation of Adult Social Care: Perpetuating a Distorted Vision?*, Bristol, Policy Press.

McNamara, B. (2001) *Fragile Lives – Death, Dying and Care*: Open University Press, Buckingham.

O'Connor, M. (2008) 'An uncertain journey: coping with transitions, survival and recurrence', in *Palliative Care Nursing- Principles and Evidence for Practice*, eds S. Payne, J. Seymour & C. Ingleton, Open University Press, Buckingham, pp. 106–120..

Payne, S. (2007) 'Living with advanced cancer', in *Handbook of Cancer Survivorship*, ed M. Feuerstein, Springer, New York, NY.

Reith, M. & Payne, M. (2009) *Social Work in End-of-life and Palliative Care*, Policy Press, Bristol.

Sekse, R.J., Raaheim, M., Blaaka, G. & Gjengedal, E. (2010) 'Life beyond Cancer: women's experiences 5 years after treatment for gynaecological cancer', *Scandinavian Journal of the Caring Sciences*, vol. 24, no. 4, pp. 799–807.

Selye, H. (1986) 'Cancer, stress and the mind', in *Cancer Stress and Death*, ed Stacey B. Day, Plenum MTdical Books, New York, NY.

Shaha, M. & Cox, C. L. (2003) 'The omnipresence of cancer', *European Journal of Oncology Nursing*, vol. 7, no. 3, pp. 191–196.

Shanfield, S.B. (1980) 'On surviving cancer: psychological considerations', *Comprehensive Psychiatry*, vol. 21, no. 2, pp. 128–134.

Small, N. (2001) 'Social work and palliative care', *British Journal of Social Work*, vol. 31, pp. 961–971.

Taylor, E. J. (1995) 'Whys and wherefores: adult patient perspectives of the meaning of cancer', *Seminars in Oncology Nursing*, vol. 11, no. 1, pp. 32–40.

Tishelman, C. & Sachs, L. (1992) 'Hopes and expectations of swedish cancer patients: contradictions surrounding patient satisfaction with care', *Psycho-Oncology*, vol. 1, no. 4, pp. 253–268.

Vachon, M. L. (2001) 'The meaning of illness to a long-term survivor', *Seminars in Oncology Nursing*, vol. 17, no. 4, pp. 279–283.

Young, E., Bury, M. & Elston, M. (1999) 'Live and/or let die : modes of social dying among women and their friends', *Mortality*, vol. 4, no. 3, pp. 269–290.

Young, E. Seale, C. & Bury, M. (1998) 'It's not like family going, is it? Negotiating friendship boundaries towards the end-of-life', *Mortality*, vol. 3, no. 1, pp. 27–43.

Lesley Adshead and Andrea Dechamps

END OF LIFE CARE: EVERYBODY'S BUSINESS

The Department of Health's End of Life Care Strategy 2008, set out ways for improving people's experience of dying in England and Wales. Hospice and specialist palliative care services were seen as having particular expertise and the strategy envisaged that their model of care should influence care in other generalist settings including social care. Palliative care social workers were identified as having knowledge and skills which could be drawn on to develop the end of life knowledge and skills of their colleagues in non-specialist settings. However, drawing on the ideas of Brown and Walter, 2013, that suggest social work has a pivotal role in remodelling hospice and palliative care, this paper examines their argument. To develop our thinking we have drawn on our experiences of sharing our expertise, through a hospice based, social work led, education and workforce development project for social care staff working in non-specialist settings.

Introduction

In this paper we critically examine the major challenges posed for end of life care in the UK with a specific focus on developing end of life care within social care services. We first consider the demographic and social context which form the key pressures for end of life care. We outline the strategic responses to these challenges, and especially the End of Life Care strategy (Department of Health, 2008) and the subsequent framework for developing the strategy within social care (NHS, 2010). The End of Life Care strategy identifies hospice and specialist palliative care services as having particular end of life care expertise and envisages that their approach should influence care provided in other non-specialist settings, including social care. In the second section we debate Brown and Walter's (2013, p. 2375) argument that this hospice and palliative care model of practice should be 'rethought' and we consider the challenge they put to social work to develop 'a more adequate model of care' — what they term a social model. We will identify where our perspectives converge and diverge. In the final part we reflect on some aspects of a workforce training and development project which builds on the hospice and palliative care model of practice. We draw on our experiences with that work to further challenge Brown and Walter's arguments. We highlight some of the important principles underpinning the hospice and palliative care model, which we feel may be at risk if the model is 'rethought' without proper attention.

By care at end of life (EOL) we are generally referring to the formal care given to those who are thought to be within the last year of life. This is the definition used in the End of Life Care Strategy (2008). For people living with reduced mental capacity, EOL needs require attention over a longer period — for these groups forward planning for EOL is crucial (CIPOLD, 2013). Brown and Walter equate formal care with paid care. However, we would not necessarily use pay as defining formal care as many people working within services providing care are volunteers drawn from the communities in which those services operate. We see *all* services — General Practitioners, district nurses, social care services, and care homes — working with people at EOL, as potentially delivering palliative care — that is holistic care focussed on the person's physical, social, psychological, and spiritual comfort and providing support for their family and other informal care givers. The professionals within these services will not usually have received accredited training in palliative care. In line with Brown and Walter, we will use the term 'hospice and palliative care' as meaning care delivered through specialist EOL care services (sometimes referred to as specialist palliative care) — though we will be questioning some of their assumptions about the nature of such services. Brown and Walter do not offer a clear definition of their 'model for practice'. We argue for a model which includes the following: desired outcomes, principles, evidence informed practice, process (strategies, methods and tools) and quality of care.

Demographic, Social and Strategic Context

Demographic pressures (ONS, 2012) are forcing policy makers to think afresh about how best to deliver health and social care services to those people approaching the EOL. Improvements in mortality rates, whilst welcome, do not necessarily represent increased years of good health; older people are frequently living with multiple chronic and degenerative conditions. Many older people are simply becoming more frail. Forty per cent of those over 85 years are assessed as having a serious disability affecting their capacity to perform activities of daily life (Centre for Population Change, 2010). The Medical Research Council Cognitive Function and Ageing Study suggest that around half a million people in England and Wales have dementia of mild or greater severity, with approximately 163,000 new cases of dementia occurring in England and Wales each year (Centre for Population Change, 2010). Many older people are living alone — 36 percent of those aged 65+ (Age UK, 2015). Some 17 percent of older people can be described as socially isolated — defined as having less than weekly contact with family, friends or neighbours (Victor *et al.*, 2003). In the same study 38 percent report some degree of loneliness. Age UK (2015) reported that 2.9 million people aged over 65 said they feel they have no one to turn to for help and support.

To address these demographic pressures and deficits identified in current EOL care, End of Life Care Strategy (Department of Health, 2008) set out a comprehensive framework for developing end of life care in England with similar strategies for the other parts of the UK. It put forward a vision of what, for many people, might be termed a 'good death' — being treated as an individual, with dignity and respect; being without pain and other symptoms; being in familiar surroundings; and being in the company of close family and/or friends (p. 9). Whilst it recognised that all settings were potentially supporting people to die well, unfortunately too many people were still dying in pain, without dignity, receiving unnecessary interventions, and in a place not of their choosing. It proposed (p. 10) a six-step pathway for delivering good care at EOL.

Both within the End of Life Care Strategy and the Social Care Framework that followed it two years later (NHS, 2010), the expertise and quality of care delivered by specialist palliative care services was recognised but the vision was for enhanced generalist services with sharing of knowledge, skills and standards from specialist services (Box 1).

BOX 1: Role and influence of Hospice and Specialist Palliative Care

Much can be learned from the holistic approach to care which has been pioneered by hospices and specialist palliative care services in this country over the past 40 years. The pioneering work of the late Dame Cicely Saunders and others has shown what can be achieved through close attention to the physical, psychological, social and spiritual needs of patients and their families. DH (2008) para 1.16

Hospices will continue to have a pivotal role within the new vision for end of life care set out in this strategy. They will continue to be centres of excellence, providing a standard of care against which other services will be measured. DH (2008) para 4.48

Palliative care social workers...have a crucial role in ensuring high quality end of life care, both within the specialist setting and within mainstream services. NHS (2010) Para 3.6

The challenge for services is laid down in the strategy — to extend the quality of care, currently available to a minority of people through hospice care, to the majority of people who will die under the care of non-specialist services including social care.

There are other visions of end of life care which see the current EOL care model as being service led and they place communities at the centre of health care — these are generally described as public health approaches (Kellehear, 2005) and make community development in relation to EOL care the priority. This has been summed up in the following way:

> In end-of-life care a community development approach involves local authorities, social services, cultural institutions and faith organizations in reflecting and responding to death, dying, loss and care. Community development in end-of-life care provides holistic approaches and changed attitudes towards the end-of life and its care (Karapliagkou and Kellehear, 2014).

Brown and Walter's Critique of Current Models of Practice in End of Life Care

Brown and Walter (2013) position their work within this public health model stressing a social response to end of life care. They challenge the social work profession in the UK 'to stake a claim and play its part in delivering EOL care' (p. 2377). They see a need for its role to be 'more clearly articulated' and thereby add their voice to many others who call on social work to play a greater role in end of life care (Holloway, 2009; Wood & Paget, 2013; College of Social Work, 2015). They fail to clarify how specialist palliative care social workers might fit into this picture.

Brown and Walter suggest current models of practice in EOL care originated from the hospice and palliative care movement. This, they suggest, was, in part, because Primary Care Trusts (who were then the lead agency for EOL Care provision), 'looked towards what they already knew for ideas and, in EOL care, it has been the palliative care movement where expertise is seen to be' (p. 2377). They describe the hospice and palliative care model — what they term the current model of practice — as being multiprofessional or hyperprofessional, with support for the patient 'almost without exception provided by the professional members of a multidisciplinary team'. They contend that this model, whilst supporting the main carer as a recipient of services in their own right, 'ignores naturally existing support networks'. They argue that social work is 'well positioned to develop a more adequate model of practice ...' (p. 2375).

They raise two key issues with this current model of practice. First they argue that the holistic hospice model of EOL practice was developed with cancer patients and claim, citing Clark (1993), that it represents 'a Rolls Royce service provided to a few' and that 'resources are unlikely to be available to expand it to everyone ...' (p. 2378). Second, they assert that the multiprofessional model can disempower as well as empower dying people and their family and friends who care for them. They acknowledge the empowering intentions behind the holistic approach of hospice and specialist palliative care services and accept that many patients have been supported to face their own deaths and their families empowered to look after them often at home (p. 2378). However, they argue, that at the same time,

> ... this approach subtly, and inherently, disempowers patients and families. It carries the clear message that dying is complex and requires skilled, multiprofessional support. In the very process of partially demedicalising dying, it further professionalises it (p. 2378–9).

Brown and Walter do not clearly state what form this professionalization takes but they do refer to its underpinning 'ideologies which presume the patient/service user to be a whole individual with a range of needs — which inevitably promotes the interests of professionals in meeting them' (p. 2379). They argue that the focus of palliative care in Western (Anglophone) societies, shaped by a discourse of individuality, has led to its emphasis on promoting choice through 'Advance Directives' and plans for 'Preferred Place of Care'. Brown and Walter suggest we should instead start with an ideology which sees 'people at the EOL as persons embedded in, and constituted by relationships' — they assert that such relationship based care is 'foreign to most of the palliative care literature' (p. 2380) and they propose an alternative model — 'a social model of end of life care that builds upon the resources and networks already surrounding individuals'. They argue that this model 'normalises dying by recognising and building upon the potential of natural networks to support families'(p. 2381). They envisage social work drawing on its 'values, culture and experience (particularly from the service user movement) to help develop these new models'. They describe the benefits of community engagement through network mobilization and suggest a 'circles of care' approach to end of life care as described by Abel *et al*. (2013). Within this approach care is provided first by resident kin (in the first circle) then from non-resident kin (the second circle), then friends, neighbours, and local community contacts, making up the outer circles. On the periphery is professional care — to be drawn on when the social network has been fully mobilised. They recognise that professionals will be needed to deliver specific services and also will be needed to empower the person's natural network, particularly for those who are network poor. Brown and Walter assert that they 'reject both a generic idealising of networks' capacities to provide support and an out-and-out dismissal of the potential of networks to support EOL care' (p. 2382).

Where We Converge

The authors of this paper are clear that a community development approach, within a public health model, can be a way forward and share much of Brown and Walter's vision; their paper is valuable in promoting both debate and practice development.

We agree that there are pressures to find new ways of working with people at EOL accepting that hospices and specialist palliative care services are never going to be able to, or indeed would wish to, directly support all people at EOL. We recognise the imperative for community development in end of life care (Kellehear, 2005, 2013; International Work Group on Death and Dying (IWG), 2014) and we see palliative and hospice care as forming a key element of such development. We agree that too often 'end of life care' has been conflated with 'end of life care *service provision*' (Karapliagkou & Kellehear, 2014, p. 9). Brown and Walter present a model for practice which, if it could be fully realized, would be helpful in ensuring that more people reach the EOL supported by those most familiar to them, and perhaps, with their networks fully mobilised, could continue to live at home for longer and be enabled to die at home if that is their wish. We are certainly at one with Brown and Walter that it is vital that care at EOL (whether delivered by family or by professionals) is based on relationships and that people's natural networks, and the confidence of those in the network are not undermined by professional practices. We are in full agreement that the social work role at EOL is poorly articulated, and that social workers across all settings bring a set of values, knowledge and skills which, if they can be drawn on fully, should enable them to play a very prominent and useful role with people at EOL and this could include network mobilisation. We also accept, though with some caveats, which we will return to later, that hospices and palliative care services have not hitherto pursued network mobilisation as a model of practice quite in the way described in Brown and Walter's paper.

Where We Diverge

Notwithstanding these areas of convergence, there are others where we would challenge Brown and Walter's assumptions which are in danger of misrepresenting the palliative care and hospice model. We would argue that social work must develop its practice in relation to EOL by taking the best that all approaches have to offer and by building close partnerships. By suggesting that social workers seek an *alternative* to the hospice and palliative care model of practice there is a danger that the proverbial baby will be thrown out with the bath water. This risk is greater if the model of palliative and hospice care is not communicated accurately and we are not persuaded that they have done this.

Brown and Walter begin their critique by referring to hospice and palliative care's roots in cancer care and by describing it as a 'Rolls Royce service provided to a few' (p. 2378). They cite a 1993 reference from Clark and fail to properly acknowledge the ways in which hospices and palliative care services have evolved since, particularly over the last decade. They assert that 'resources are unlikely to be available to expand it to everyone requiring services at this stage' (p. 2378). They do not define what they mean by 'requiring services at this stage' but it was never part of the EOLC strategy to see hospice and palliative care provide services directly to all dying people — this would clearly be a misallocation of specialist resources. Certainly we would not try to argue that access to specialist palliative care is equitable, for many studies have found that people in areas of highest deprivation, marginalised groups, some BAME groups, people with non-malignant conditions, the oldest old, and people with dementia and learning disabilities have all been less than well served (Tuffrey-Wijne et al., 2007; Oliviere et al., 2011; Dixon et al., 2015). Specialist services must seek better ways of delivering their care so that these inequities are significantly reduced, and there is evidence that there are many initiatives underway to address this (Calanzani et al., 2013). However, as Dixon et al. (2015) point out, many dying people are not receiving palliative care of any kind — from either specialists or generalists. Hughes-Hallett et al. (2011) suggest that this is true of about 92,000 people in England each year. In a report for Age UK, Harrop (2011) estimates more broadly that 800,000 people a year would benefit from elderly care but do not receive it from any professional source. Thus many of these people are approaching the EOL with unmet needs, both physical and psychosocial.

Our fear is that by continuing to portray the hospice and palliative care model of practice as something rather fixed and exclusive, rather than by acknowledging that it is a constantly evolving model adapting to current challenges (see for example Richardson, 2012), Brown and Walter's paper could, perhaps unwittingly, lead social workers to imagine that the palliative and hospice care model has nothing to offer for the majority.

We concur that the current model of EOL care tends towards a top down, service led provision but in their paper Brown and Walter appear to take their critique a step beyond this and describe a 'doing to' approach in the hospice and palliative care model with the agenda being set by the professional.

In this multiprofessional model, support for the patient is almost without exception provided by the professional members of a multidisciplinary team, whether it be a community nurse teaching the family carer about lifting and handling or a social worker advising about stress and family dynamics (p. 2378).

We would suggest that this is one 'reading' of the hospice and palliative care approach but research carried out by one of the authors with users of hospice and palliative care social work services (Beresford *et al.*, 2007) would point to there being other, possibly more nuanced, readings about how expertise and, indeed, authority might be handled within hospice and palliative care (Box 2).

Box 2: Quotes from service users of hospice and palliative care social work

'She was there and she was just there to listen to me and I was the one that did most of the talking and I kind of led the actual meeting.' (Woman patient, age group 56-65)

'The strengths were that there was somebody there to listen to you and to help you, yeah listen, not advise you.' (Bereaved man, age unknown)

'Just when I needed it she took control...' (Bereaved woman age group 26-35)

'I depended on the social worker because I was very, very weak ...I couldn't make my own decisions ....I trusted her...she explained everything to me so that in my weaker state I never, ever doubted her (Woman patient, age group 80+)

(Beresford et al 2007)

As acknowledged earlier, it is accepted, with some caveats, that network mobilisation has not always been pursued in the way that Brown and Walters envisage. We accept this, in the sense that a community development, public health approach has not always been at the forefront of the hospice and palliative approach to practice. However, this has been changing rapidly and there are many current examples of hospice led initiatives, which seek to extend their role, taking on a health promotion dimension through community engagement — working with schools, local community groups, and volunteers attached to the hospice — to develop awareness of death and dying, encourage conversations about death and dying, and building compassionate communities (Richardson, 2012; Kellehear, 2013; International Work Group on Death and Dying (IWG), 2014). Paul and Sallow (2013) found that sixty percent of hospices engaged in initiatives of this kind.

Of greater concern still is Brown and Walter's assertion that hospice and palliative care 'ignores naturally existing support networks'. This seems to us, as long-standing professionals in hospice and palliative care, to be far from our understanding of our approach. It is telling to look back at some of the writings of Dame Cicely Saunders, the founder of the modern hospice movement (Box 3).

> **Box 3: Quotes from Dame Cicely Saunders on hospice care**
>
> *'All the work of the professional team, the skilled symptom control, the supportive nursing **and the mobilisation of community resources** are to enable the dying person to live until he dies, at his own maximum potential, performing to the limit of his physical activity and mental capacity, with control and independence wherever possible. If he is recognised as the unique person he is and **helped to live as part of his family and in other relationships** he can still reach out to his hopes and expectations and to what has the deepest meaning for him and end his life with a sense of completion.'*
>
> (From On Dying Well, first published in The Cambridge Review 27 Feb 1984 pp49-52 Reproduced in Cicely Saunders Selected Writings 1958-2004 Oxford University Press 2006)
>
> *We began to look at **the whole family unit** and the support needed to enable them to remain as **the most important part of the caring team**.*
>
> (Taken from DCS Templeton Prize Speech. May 1981 Reproduced in Selected Writings)

It could be argued that this vision has since been diluted, with the focus now more squarely on the provision of direct care for the individual through the members of the multi-disciplinary team. We dispute this, as this statement from a briefing paper of the National Council of Palliative Care illustrates :

The social fabric of their lives is central to how they make sense of their illness experiences, the meanings they draw upon to understand these and the range of resources they can call upon to help them manage them (Field, 2000).

What Brown and Walter describe as their new model of practice is, we would argue, often what already happens in practice,

… health and social care professionals become part of the dying person's/carer's team, providing paid services where more naturally occurring unpaid forms of care run out … Often they turn for help with specific tasks, rather than for holistic care. Professionals who understand this model see their role partly as delivering specific services, but also partly as helping to empower the person's natural network (p. 2381).

There are still, nevertheless, certain significant deficits in EOL care which they do not fully address — the dying phase not recognised, conversations never initiated, late planning, and choices not known and so not honoured. They do not address the individual fears and anxieties about death which hinder identification of the dying phase and inhibit conversations, both for family and social networks, and for professionals. The circles of care approach which they advocate, if interpreted clumsily, could heighten the risk of bringing in professionals only at the end — much as palliative care has often been said to be brought in 'too late' — a hazard both for planning and the quality of care itself.

Brown and Walter fail to develop their critique in relation to many of the thorny issues — network poverty, issues of risk, and especially the complexity and technicality of end of life care, even in what might be termed 'straightforward' deaths. They claim that the hospice and palliative care model is both empowering and 'inherently disempowering'. While informal carers and, indeed, generalist health and social care staff can feel de-skilled in the face of apparent 'expert' knowledge this need not be an automatic thing. It can be avoided if people build partnerships at an individual and organisational level where there can be more of a mutual exchange with all sides contributing to, and drawing from, the total stock of knowledge, insight and experience.

Throughout Brown and Walter's paper there is a tendency for the complexities of EOL care, especially the physical, to be skimmed over. Families and communities in history may have coped but we would suggest expectations were significantly lower, protection from risk was not so prominent on the national or personal agenda, and most importantly, people tended to die more quickly with fewer co-morbidities. Within palliative care and other health services a whole raft of strategies, tools and skills have developed for providing optimal physical care — to relieve pain and other complex and troubling symptoms such as nausea, breathlessness and fatigue, to preserve skin integrity, to help with anxiety and agitation, to manage catheters, to manage fluid and nutritional needs, and so on. End of life care now is often very technical. This is not to say that family members and others in the network do not have, or cannot learn skills over time, but inevitably it will be professionals who take the lead in supporting them to do this — and today it is often the specialists in hospice and palliative care services who have developed the greatest expertise in using these skills, specifically with people at EOL. It is paramount, therefore, that there is close integration of informal and formal care networks.

We believe that if Brown and Walter's ideas are to be capitalised on — if social workers are going to develop their role in end of life care and support people to identify and mobilise their networks — then first some additional 'building blocks' of skills, knowledge, and confidence, will need to be put in place. These are currently found most frequently — though not exclusively — in hospice and palliative care services. By building partnerships and drawing strands of the two models closer together we suggest that end of life care can only benefit whether it be delivered informally through social networks or more formally through generalist and specialist services. This blended approach is what we have been aiming for in a workforce development and training initiative and it is to this that we now turn.

Putting Our Vision into Practice

The project is run from St Christopher's Hospice in SE London and has been coordinated and delivered by the authors of this paper, both palliative care social workers, along with other colleagues. As a hospice-led project, it lies within the model of practice that Brown and Walter suggest is over professionalised, neglectful of, and inherently disempowering to, people's social relationships and networks. These are strong charges; we draw on some of our experiences within this project to demonstrate how we can work within our own model but nevertheless work in a way that is compatible with, and supportive of, the community development approach advocated by Brown and Walter and others.

This project was initially funded by the National End of Life Care Programme, as a test site, for the implementation of *'Supporting People to live and die well: a framework for social care at the end of life* (NHS, 2010). More recently this training has been commissioned by the local authorities concerned. The project illustrates one of the ways that hospice and palliative care has been encouraged, with government backing, to share expertise with non-specialist colleagues. Our guiding philosophy is that end of life care is everybody's business — too important to be left to hospices. The key message within our training is that EOL is not the preserve of experts; we can, and must, all play a part.

The project focuses on building partnerships with local authorities and working with them to develop EOL awareness and skills of their own social care staff — in the main social workers. The partnerships with local authorities have also enabled us to reach many other community based services as the local authority training and development is generally opened up to their partner organisations. To give some examples: services that support people with learning disabilities; local Alzheimer's groups; community BAME groups; mental health organisations; supported housing services; voluntary sector day centres and healthy living centres. Most of the professionals we have met through this work are regularly working with people approaching the EOL but frequently do not feel they have a role to play.

We work at three levels: first with senior and service managers; second with social workers and others designated as the EOL lead for their team; and third, with all other staff. We have run many courses and carried out many visits to different teams and organisations. We have no space here to go into detail but whatever the level, and the nature of the specific training, we find there are some key elements that form the cornerstones of our approach to sharing our expertise and we depict these in Figure 1. Undoubtedly these are the building blocks that would be needed to take Brown and Walter's vision forward. In the following section of the paper we address each of the building blocks depicted in Figure 1 and show some of the ways we have incorporated them into our training.

Raising Awareness and Developing Compassionate Communities and Professionals

It has been a conscious decision that, where possible, courses should be taught at the hospice, arguably the best way to raise awareness. Taking people on a tour so that they can see for themselves what the atmosphere is like, has clearly dispelled fears, mis-

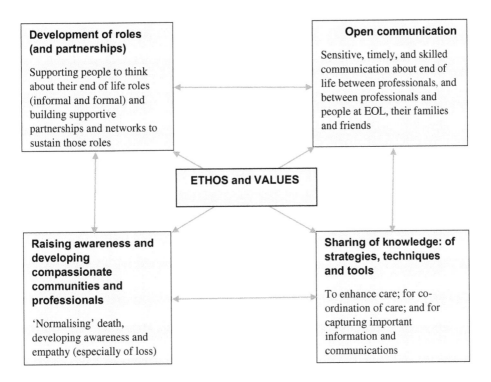

FIGURE 1   Key elements of our training and development initiative.

apprehensions and sometimes prejudices about palliative care. We see people relax as they are shown around and as they mix with patients and families in the social space. They often comment on how it is 'life' that is so evident rather than 'death' and how healthy living and quality of life are being promoted in the face of death — through the surrounding ambience, and the gardens, the busyness of the rehabilitation gym, and the sense of creativity in the art and photography produced by patients, families and the local community. They have the chance to see that St Christopher's opens its doors and welcomes the public not just as volunteers or as potential fundraisers (though these are an undeniable part of community involvement) but on a more routine basis — to a curry night, to the community choir, the quilting group, and Sunday lunch, to mention just a few instances. They see evidence of partnerships with other organisations such as care homes, colleges, and local arts organisations. If they encounter one of the many visiting school groups and see the children and young people interacting with patients and families and learning first-hand about living with life limiting illness, they can see how the hospice is actively playing its part in 'normalising dying' and building healthy and resilient communities for the future. They will see pictures on the wall showing some of our young volunteers from a local performing arts school enjoying the time they spend with teenagers and young people, living with life limiting illness, who attend our young people's project.

Some course participants admit they were nervous before they arrived. They felt they would be confronted with death in an unsettling way. We certainly do not avoid mention of death — there are information leaflets all around — on all aspects of EOL

— physical, social, spiritual, and emotional. We do not avoid sadness and loss, which finds its expression in some of the art work on the walls and in the books left open in the Pilgrim Room (our quiet space for use by people of all faiths or none). These books offer patients, family and friends the chance to write messages, poems, and memories, and are well used. Sadness and grief are not concealed but neither do they dominate. People always seem more animated and engaged with the training after the tour. The tour also allows us to explain the structure of our service with its elements of self-management, community based care, in-patient care, and bereavement care — the in-patient care generally having a much lower profile than most of the course participants expect and there is much effort to re-emphasise the social.

The tour of the hospice is, we believe, very powerful in demonstrating how the traditional hospice and palliative care model — with its respect for dying people and their families, its open acceptance of death as a normal part of life, its emphasis on holistic multi-disciplinary care, and its emphasis on 'living until you die' — can be blended successfully with the evolving public health oriented model of care with its focus on partnerships, community engagement, and on developing compassionate communities. The tour affords participants a taste of the ethos and values underpinning hospice and palliative care.

Raising awareness of death is a key part of our training. We want to support individuals to become compassionate professionals — essential if they are to play a part in developing a social model of end of life care. Many of our courses include content on loss and change, together with coping and resilience. We focus on loss both as a dominant theme at EOL and as an element ever present in all branches of social work and social care; new skills will always be relevant and transferable. Despite this familiarity with loss, it was clear that in their day-to-day practice, many of them shy away from conversations about death. They do not automatically retain confidence in their generic skills — they say they lack the time for in-depth work; they fear they will cause distress; they have concern that the subject might be culturally sensitive or taboo, and they worry that talking about death will awaken their own anxieties and memories.

We believe it is vital to provide an opportunity for participants to really 'drill down' into the idea of loss. Most people reaching EOL will have experienced multiple losses, as well as some gains, but we find that many social care workers and social workers have little or no professionally sanctioned opportunities for reflecting on such issues. They rapidly move to thoughts about practical needs, and how these can be met. We offer space for them to think through the countless losses and changes encountered at EOL — and in so doing, we would suggest course participants become more attuned to, and more empathetic to, the real experiences of people facing the EOL. Much of our reflection is then about losses of relationships, networks, and community involvement, and about loss of identity and self-esteem.

We are not suggesting that the majority of these professionals lack awareness or empathy but we have been told that such traits and qualities can become blunted in jobs that are frequently highly time constrained, and where the imperative is to keep focussed on the task immediately at hand whether that be assessment, review, brokerage or the provision of direct hands-on care. Administrative roles, such as determining eligibility, can crowd out opportunities for reflective social work that calls for social workers to more fully use themselves. A comment we have heard numerous times is that properly engaging with EOL work, 'makes me feel like a social worker again'.

Development of Roles and Partnerships

It should be clear that our project rests on building new partnerships with local authorities and with other organisations. We see this project not simply as being about delivering commissioned training but about establishing and developing links and relationships
with community colleagues that can be sustained over time. It is about getting to know
and understand the real challenges that these colleagues face. We have already referred
to the difficulties some social care staff face in identifying their role in relation to end of
life care. We accept that this may, in part, be because of the dominance of health services
in EOL care but it is arguably more complex and closely linked to the way services are
structured and funded. Usually social workers are well trained, though not necessarily
in end of life care, and eager to develop their EOL care role but struggle to develop their
practice within an unwieldy structure. They are able to offer little continuity of care —
support is fragmented and people's care is passed from team to team, which limits the
likelihood of building the rapport and relationships that end of life care need; though
we have observed many attempts to overcome these obstacles. Before social workers
can take up the challenges Brown and Walter identify they will need to have much more
scope to practise social work in a less constrained way. Others have made the same
observations about social work with older people (Milne *et al.*, 2014). Our aim within
the project has been to provide as many opportunities as possible for social workers to
critically examine their roles — to identify where they *can* make a difference within all
the constraining factors; even small changes should be celebrated. We have realised that
conversely staff and volunteers working in various community organisations are often
working at a more grassroots level with close involvement of local people, sometimes
at a decision-making level, and have often built very solid and long term relationships
with the people they support. Such organisations may be an important part of an older
or ill person's social network. However staff, especially volunteers, have often received
little training and sometimes therefore underestimate their role and their skills. By
offering some formal training and mentoring we have been able to encourage organisations to take on EOL (and bereavement) issues in an enhanced way. One example is
a community centre that has introduced advance care planning conversations alongside
its wellbeing assessments of older people, making conversations about EOL routine and
linked to healthy living rather than disease. After some initial training and support from
us they have worked out how they can best put this into action within their context,
taking into account their particular service users, with their social and cultural needs,
and have gone on to train their own volunteers without our direct involvement.

Open Communication

Open, and timely communication, which is sensitive to diversity and cultural difference,
lies at the heart of good end of life care and is a constant theme in our training initiative.
Many of the people we work with have the skills, but lack the confidence to fully utilise
them in relation to EOL. If they are going to work with people at EOL to mobilise their
networks, honest communication which does not avoid or skim over the potential difficulties, is needed. We provide many opportunities for practice and for discussion on

barriers to effective communication. We offer practice on initiating EOL conversations, responding to cues, and on having challenging conversations. We have shadowed some workers, at their request, to observe and reflect with them on their practice.

Sharing of Knowledge: of Strategies, Techniques and Tools

We have concentrated on sharing the EOL tools which we feel have the potential to promote, enhance, or record communication about EOL issues. These include 'Gold Standards Framework' and End of Life Registers, 'Coordinate My Care', Advance Care Plans, and 'Priorities for Care of the Dying Person' (see http://www.goldstandards-framework.org.uk/library-tools-amp-resources). Most of the social care professionals have only the scantiest information about such tools and resources and this is probably because most of these have originated from health care settings which have not always been effective in involving social care colleagues or ensuring that different electronic systems could support the same tools. Funding structures for end of life care have also clouded the picture. The majority of the tools encourage recognition that EOL (or loss of capacity) could be approaching; support early planning for EOL; promote open communication and improve coordination of care. Although they were perhaps health driven in the first instance they are all relevant for social care. If social workers are to develop confidence in their EOL role and certainly if they are to develop new social models for EOL care it is vital that they are able to fully engage in conversations and collaborations with health colleagues.

We have only been able to share a little of the experience we have gained from our training initiative, but hope we have demonstrated some of the beliefs and values that underpin that work and the key elements that have driven it forward. Certainly we have found that both local authority social workers and other professionals working in a variety of organisations are keen to develop their awareness, role, skills and confidence in end of life care. The main challenge, for us and them, has been to find ways of taking this work forward in an environment where pressures on resources constrain local authorities, and threaten to further erode the existing, limited, role that social workers have in working with people at EOL. We are constantly adapting our approach to try and find ways that we can, together, overcome some of these hurdles.

Conclusion

Significant demographic challenges are posed for the development of EOL care in the UK and social care services and social workers must play a major role in this development. Brown and Walter (2013) have challenged social work to develop a social model which would prioritise the mobilisation and support of informal networks to support the dying person. They have critiqued the current hospice and palliative approach as overly professional, inherently disempowering, and as failing to take account of people's naturally occurring social networks.

There is much in their paper which we support: the importance of developing and enhancing the social work role; the need to support and not undermine informal networks at EOL and the value of relationship based care. However we have argued that aspects of Brown and Walter's depiction of the hospice and palliative care model are somewhat of a caricature, and some of their arguments are dated, as they fail to acknowledge, or take account of, recent developments in palliative care which stress partnership working and community engagement. We have also argued that they fail to grapple with some of the thorny issues that make end of life care so challenging, in particular the complexity of much end of life care.

Most importantly, they have described their model as alternative to, rather than complementary to, the hospice and palliative care model (p. 2381). We disagree. All of us — professionals and ordinary citizens — have a part to play in end of life care, and partnership working, integration, and mutual respect is essential if this is to happen. Complementarity is necessary, with the best from the hospice and palliative care approach *and* the community development models informing future practice.

Disclosure statement

No potential conflict of interest was reported by the authors.

References

Abel, J., Walter, T., Carey, L. B., Rosenberg, J., Noonan, K., Horsfall, D., Leonard, R., Rumbold, B. & Morris, D. (2013) 'Circles of care: should community development redefine the practice of palliative care?', *BMJ Supportive Palliative Care*, vol. 2, no. 1, pp. 129–133.

Age UK. (2015) *Later Life in the United Kingdom, Age UK Factsheet April 2015*. Available at http://www.ageuk.org.uk/Documents/EN-GB/Factsheets/Later_Life_UK_factsheet.pdf [accessed 22 April 2015].

Beresford, P., Adshead, L. & Croft, S. (2007) *Palliative Care, Social Work and Service Users: Making Life Possible*, Jessica Kingsley, London.

Brown, L. & Walter, T. (2013) 'Towards a social model of end-of-life care', *British Journal of Social Work*, vol. 44, no. 8, pp. 2375–2390.

Calanzani, N., Higginson, I. J. & Gomes, B. (2013) *Current and Future Needs for Hospice Care: An Evidence-based Report*, Help the Hospices.

Centre for Population Change. (2010) *Demographic Issues, Projections and Trends: Older People with High Support Needs in the UK*, Joseph Rowntree Foundation. Available at http://www.jrf.org.uk/sites/files/jrf/high-support-needs-demographic-issues.pdf [accessed 22 April 2015].

CIPOLD. (2013) *The confidential inquiry into premature deaths of people with learning disabilities (CIPOLD)*, Norah Fry Research Centre, University of Bristol. Available at http://www.bristol.ac.uk/media-library/sites/cipold/migrated/documents/fullfinalreport.pdf [accessed 4 May 2015].

College of Social Work. (2015) 'The route to success in end of life care — achieving quality for social work'. Available at www.nhsiq.nhs.uk/download.ashx?mid=8190&nid=8189 [accessed 18 August 2015].

Department of Health. (2008) *End of Life Care Strategy — Promoting High Quality Care for all Adults at the End of Life*, Crown, London.

Dixon, J., King, D., Matosevic, T., Clark, M. & Knapp, M. (2015) 'Equity in the provision of palliative care in the UK: review of evidence'. Available at www.pssru.ac.uk/publication-details.php?id=4962 [accessed 22 April 2015].

Field, D. (2000) *What Do We Mean by Psychosocial? Briefing Paper No 4, March*, National Council for Palliative Care, London.

Harrop, A. (2011) *Care in Crisis: Causes and Solutions*. Age UK. Available at www.ageuk.org.uk/professional-resources [accessed 24 April 2015].

Holloway, M. (2009) 'Dying old in the twenty-first century: a neglected issue for social work', *International Social Work*, vol. 53, no. 5, pp. 1–13.

Hughes-Hallett, T., Craft, A. & Davies, C. (2011) *Palliative Care Funding Review: Funding the Right Care and Support for Everyone*, Department of Health, London.

International Work Group on Death and Dying (IWG). (2014) 'A call to action: an IWG charter for a public health approach to dying, death, and loss', *Omega*, vol. 69, no. 4, pp. 401–420.

Karapliagkou, A. & Kellehear, A. (2014) *Public Health Approaches to End of Life Care: A Toolkit*, Public Health England and the National Council or Palliative Care, London.

Kellehear, A. (2005) *Compassionate Cities: Public Health and End of Life Care*, Routledge, London.

Kellehear, A. (2013) 'Compassionate communities: end-of-life care as everyone's responsibility', *QJM*, vol. 106, no. 12, pp. 1071–1075.

Milne, A., Sullivan, M. P., Tanner, D., Richards, S., Ray, M., Lloyd, L., Beech, C. & Phillips, J. (2014) *Social Work with Older People: A Vision for the Future*, The College of Social Work, London.

NHS. (2010) *Supporting People to Live and Die Well: A Framework for Social Care at the End of Life. Report of the Social Care Advisory Group of the National End of Life Care Programme*, Crown, London.

Oliviere, D., Monroe, B. & Payne, S. (eds.) (2011) *Death, Dying, and Social Differences*, 2nd ed., Oxford University Press, Oxford.

ONS. (2012) Population Ageing in the United Kingdom, Its Constituent Countries and the European Union. Available at http://www.ons.gov.uk/ons/dcp171776_258607.pdf [accessed 22 April 2015].

Paul, S. & Sallnow, L. (2013) 'Public health approaches to end-of-life care in the UK: an online survey of palliative care services', *BMJ Supportive and Palliative Care*, vol. 3, pp. 196–199.

Richardson, H. (2012) 'A public health approach to palliative care in East London', in *International Perspectives on Public Health and Palliative Care*, pp. 110–122, eds L. Sallnow, S. Kumar & A. Kellehear, Routledge, London.

Tuffrey-Wijne, I., McEnhill, L., Curfs, L. & Hollins, S. (2007) 'Palliative care provision for people with intellectual disabilities: interviews with specialist palliative care professionals in London', *Palliative Medicine*, vol. 21, no. 6, pp. 493–499.

Victor, C., Bowling, A., Bond, J. & Scambler, S. (2003) *Loneliness, Social Isolation and Living Alone in Later Life, Research Findings: 17*, Growing Older Programme, Economic and Social Research Council, Sheffield.

Wood, C. & Paget, A. (2013) *'People's Final Journey Must Be One of Their Choosing ...' Ways and Means*, report published by Demos, London, 18 June.

Rebecca Chaddock

INTEGRATING EARLY MULTI-DISCIPLINARY ADVANCE CARE PLANNING INTO CORE SOCIAL WORK PRACTICE: SOCIAL WORKERS' BREAD AND BUTTER

Many people remain unaware of their rights under the Mental Capacity Act, 2005 to make plans in advance and often approach the end of their lives without being asked about their thoughts and preferences by family or professionals. The author argues that in order for all citizens to attain their preferences at end of life, it is imperative that there is cross professional, organisational and operational agreement, paperwork and a shared understanding of Advanced Care Planning (ACP) that advocates early intervention. Skilled communication is the bedrock of social work, and difficult conversations are a routine part of daily practice. Integrating ACP into general social work practice offers a congruent approach to introducing ACP at an early stage. Drawing on the author's experience of implementing a county wide ACP project in Cumbria, this paper will advocate a standardised approach across health and social care with social work as a key tenet.

Introduction

Addressing end-of-life care in the UK involves tackling an increasingly complex set of issues that form one of the major challenges to health and social care provision in this country. The impact on the provision of palliative care by societal change is significant; we are living longer, and doing so with increasing levels of frailty, disability and chronic health conditions (Gomes & Higginson, 2008). Most deaths in the UK are of people in older age and from cardio-vascular or respiratory disease (Office of National Statistics, 2014). It is not a straightforward picture however; numbers of people diagnosed with dementia are increasing year on year (Department of Health, 2009; Prince *et al.*, 2014) and people with life limiting illnesses are living longer. In addition there are other factors to consider such as the range of health problems leading to early death for homeless people (Thomas, 2012), and that a significant proportion of the prison population now have end-of-life care needs (Prisons and Probation Ombudsman, 2014). Inevitably, different and more protracted illness trajectories challenge traditional models of social care as well as palliative care services.

For some time there has been a consensus about the need to improve the quality of end-of-life care in the UK, but the process of doing so is far from simple. There is often a disconnect between the policy makers, professionals delivering care, and the people receiving care as their health deteriorates, and there may be a number of reasons for this. British society is generally poor at acknowledging that death is a reality and most people avoid talking about the practicalities that surround it. It is therefore unsurprising that the majority are often ill-equipped and unprepared when it happens (Gawande, 2014). Priorities and preferences are not routinely elicited from people until they are dying, by which point decisions can be a 'needs must' compromise rather than a carefully considered, empowered choice. Beginning to address this question therefore requires significant societal and cultural adjustment. It involves a multi professional commitment from every sector of health and social care across both statutory and voluntary sectors, as well as from commissioners and policy makers (Barclay & Forrest, 2007) and a coordinated approach that is clearly and consistently communicated to the general public.

In 2005 Hans Clausen and colleagues observed that palliative and end-of-life care has been seen as an issue of 'health' in which social work has been conspicuous by its absence, and ten years on little has changed. However, the relatively small numbers of social workers practising exclusively within palliative care find that people's experience of terminal illness is complex, demanding a holistic appreciation of the person in their family and community context (APCSW, 2016; Hughes, Firth and Oliviere, 2014 and 2015). After addressing immediate physical needs, patients' overriding concerns are often for people that are important to them and family members, or how to pay the bills, or how to stay 'me' while grappling with what it means to have lost the 'future' they and those around them had taken for granted.

In light of this, it is predictable that in legislating, the government emphasise integration and partnership working across health and social care. In England and Wales, the wellbeing principle underpins the legislation (Care Act, 2014), and across the Union, practitioners are required by law to provide personalised care and support, allow continuity of care across areas, and act to promote prevention. Since 2005, the Mental Capacity Act has provided a statutory framework to both empower and protect people in England who may not be able to make their own decisions (Mental Capacity Act, 2005). The rights enshrined in the Act relate to assessment of capacity, best interests and provision for advance planning into a time when capacity may be lost. In the context of palliative care, Advance Care Planning (ACP) has long been considered 'best practice' (National End of Life Care Programme, 2012) and has been shown to improve outcomes of end-of-life care, patient experience and family satisfaction (Detering et al., 2010). Despite this, it has not become a standard part of professional practice outside specialist palliative and hospice care.

Deciding Right and advance care planning

Over the last five years, a committed group of varied professionals in the north have collaboratively produced a framework that aims to address this. The 'Deciding Right' framework was developed under the leadership of Claud Regnard, Consultant in Palliative Medicine (St Oswald's Hospice and Newcastle upon Tyne Hospitals NHS Foundation Trust). The Deciding Right development group recognised that to attain preferences at end of life, a joined-up, standardised approach was required with agreement across professional, organisational and operational boundaries — a shared vision grounded in shared documentation for people in the last year of life. The framework (Northern England Strategic Clinical Networks, 2012) brings together advance care planning, cardiopulmonary resuscitation decisions, and emergency healthcare plans, ensuring compliance with both national guidelines and legislation. Deciding Right provides clear principles for all healthcare organisations and professionals to follow, focusing end-of-life care decisions on the individual patient's needs and wishes, rather than organisational policies and procedures. Under the framework, it is every professional's responsibility to inform patients of their right to make choices about future care, to talk to them about their wishes, to support them to record these on the appropriate documentation, and to share the forms appropriately. The standardised Deciding Right documentation captures preferences, wishes and decisions and should be recognised by all health and social care professionals. The documentation belongs to the person, and while copies are disseminated to the professional team, the originals are kept in a yellow folder which can be taken with them wherever they go. This allows the person to be at the centre and in control of their own planning for the future and enables an ongoing conversation to take place over multiple settings and with different professionals as their illness progresses. It is believed that effective implementation of Deciding Right will play a part in minimising the likelihood of unnecessary or unwanted treatment and care, reducing unnecessary hospital admissions and in ensuring that people who are likely to lose capacity are able to continue to influence and direct their care.

The embodiment of Deciding Right in Cumbria grew from an acknowledgment that in order to improve end-of-life care for all patients and those close to them and indeed for all people in receipt of services not just those in the last year of life, a change of culture was required within both health and social care. The commissioners recognised that this must incorporate a practical roll-out on the ground as well as an overarching strategic commitment. The Cumbrian project has proactively included social work in the core professional target group, and this has been key in moving ACP forwards across the county. The central tenet of the Cumbrian roll-out of training is that all citizens with capacity have a right to make decisions about their future, and that in order to record decisions on documentation, it is often the conversation around choices that matters most. Consequently, training and information resources have been developed for professionals, people in receipt of services, and the general public. The public information leaflet firmly establishes this as 'for everyone', and approaches the subject from the perspective of rights and choices about the future without mentioning death or dying. In this way people can bring their own context to the non threatening introduction to advance care planning and follow the signposting to further information if they wish. Feedback suggests that this approach has helped people begin to think through what is important to them, come to an understanding of what they might want to refuse and who they need to involve in the process, and to complete the paperwork that enables this to happen (Chaddock *et al.*, 2014). Deciding Right in Cumbria has provided a clear structure that facilitates improved communication with individuals, but also between professionals. For example there is currently a programme of work being undertaken with Care Homes, GPs and District Nurses, in order to better understand each other's roles, facilitate better communication, encourage collaboration, and provide more effective and responsive care for residents. Whilst the full success of the Deciding Right project in the county is unlikely to be seen for some years, early signs are that the people of Cumbria have greatly increased access to advance care planning conversations, are discussing their preferences and choices with professionals and are recording these on the recognised regional forms.

Challenges

Attempting an ambitious programme of change on this scale has not been without difficulties and the initial challenge was securing the pan-Cumbria agreement that this was the way forward. There is always a danger, in taking a standardised approach to address a complex set of problems over a diverse and competing health and social care economy, that the outcome will inevitably be too generic to be meaningful. The documentation is standardized and used in every setting. Therefore, in establishing that the conversation with the individual is the pinnacle and aim of the approach, the forms themselves become the vehicle for recording the person's choices and decisions, rather than the ultimate goal. In hindsight, it is clear that to have spent more time in the early stages embedding the documentation into the electronic systems would have been enormously beneficial; rather than every professional group becoming frustrated by the practicalities, facilitators could have concentrated more on the shared approach and early intervention. It is recognised that a truly shared record and multi professional working across health and social care requires much more integrated and robust IT systems and protocols than are currently in operation. Another charge often levelled at the project is that the public need to be better informed before they come to talk to professionals about advance planning, as they often begin with little notion of what it is, what it involves or what they would like. The conversations are ongoing in Cumbria about how to better involve the public with their right to make decisions about their future care, and about what that might entail.

Making this conversation a priority at diagnosis for people with dementia has been an area where the project has yet to make inroads. In this context it can be argued that the conversations are just too big, that they require people to confront the reality of what is happening to them before they are ready, and this is a concern. However, social workers understand instinctively the power imbalance present in working with vulnerable people, and the profession has much to offer in supporting heath to address some of these issues. Professionals often have knowledge, understanding and experience of what is likely to happen in the course of someone's illness progression that is not shared by the person or those around them. Although it is often a professional judgement about how far to press conversations of this nature, it is difficult to justify withholding the opportunity to have an informed discussion from people with dementia as they come to terms with and think through their changed circumstances. Social workers consider people in their familial and social context, and this often has much to offer in engaging people in thinking through the future, not just for individuals, but for all those affected (APCSW, 2016). Enabling people who are facing a future of deteriorating cognitive function and a life that will eventually be out of their control, to talk through their right to make decisions about their future care, can enable them to regain some of the control and plan for the life they will go on to live. It can be argued that at heart this is an issue of social justice that tackles health inequalities, and one that is not just about cognitive function. In a poignant address to a professional group, the husband of a young woman with MND said: 'I wish we'd known how important practising with the communication aid was. All those afternoons when we just enjoyed being together, watching telly. Now we can see it because it's just so difficult to understand what she wants now, … and I suppose people said it back then, but we didn't know what we were saying no to.' The issue of informed consent is well established, but in a sense it is the conversations around 'informed refusal' that are at issue here. It is a well sung refrain in the Deciding Right sessions that people can decide not to have in-depth conversations about their future, but they must understand their right is to do so, and that it is part of the professionals' duty of care to continue to offer opportunities for them to talk later.

From the Cumbrian project we are learning that conversations about 'the future' need to start much earlier. It has been interesting to observe that, despite much professional anxiety, there has been a clear appetite from the general public to engage with the project. At one Patient Participation Group session on a stormy November evening, five or six people were expected for the 'Getting your affairs in order' session. From the usual advert in the practice, over seventy people turned up and the practice manager had to relocate the session to the school. Some had heard about it from family members, some had travelled over 25 miles, three generations of one family came to hear about it together, and everyone had a story to tell. Most people used words like 'horrific', 'barbaric', and 'terrible' to describe what happened to someone they knew and they all wanted 'to make sure nothing like that ever happens to me or mine'. There was not one piece of information left that night; people even took the examples that were stuck to the stand. Engaging people with advance care planning positively before they face a terminal illness enables a very different conversation to take place, and one which becomes part of the rich tapestry of life rather than death.

This reflects the growing move towards public health approaches in palliative care (Kellehear, 2005; Paul, 2013) and it has been exciting to see how well this has been received in Cumbria, even in the small way that we have begun. By the time people have come to terms with a dementia diagnosis or come into palliative care services, they have often already lost something of their sense of agency and often feel swept along. One lady commented during her husband's palliative chemotherapy: 'It feels like we're being dragged around a roller coaster by the disease, we're out of control and at the same time are terrified about what'll happen when it stops.' We have found that it is possible to help people to live the way that they choose right up until they die, but achieving this requires society broaching difficult conversations with honesty, clear thinking time, energy and planning on the part of the person, their family and those close to them, and for health and social care professionals. Sadly, the majority of people approach the end of their lives without ever being asked about their thoughts, wishes and preferences, missing out on the opportunity to take or regain control of the roller coaster.

Communication: a social worker's bread and butter

Social workers are already agents of change for individuals, families, communities and wider society (APCSW, 2016), and difficult conversations are social workers' bread and butter. They frequently enter people's lives in moments of crisis and have a key role in enabling individuals and their families to adapt by taking control of their lives, so they can continue to live as independently and autonomously as possible. Community teams often support people through incurable illness for years before they come under the remit of specialist palliative care (Draper *et al.*, 2013). It can be argued therefore, that social workers are ideally placed to introduce people to their rights under law and help them think about what would be important for them. The skill set required in order to introduce complicated concepts and troubling realities is already an integral part of social work practice; reality rarely lives up to expectation in social care. Assisting people to make contingency plans for an anticipated emergency or recurrent problem is standard practice. Widening this to include a broader conversation about the person's right to make choices about their future would make a significant difference to their ability to direct their care. The importance and benefit of doing this is evident in working with people with dementia, but the principle extends to all people accessing social work services.

A high level of skill is required for this kind of discussion, as it has the potential for significant psychosocial impact because of its relevance to a person's sense of identity. For any of us, to lose something that defines a part of who we are, how we see ourselves and want others to see us, would require significant adjustment and may result in significant distress. People with a palliative illness often experience a progressive loss of meaning as their condition worsens and their health declines towards the ultimate loss of identity, death itself (Yalom, 2008). It is not difficult to imagine how empowering and reassuring it could be to talk to someone about how you see yourself, what is important for you, to be encouraged tell decision makers what you want, and how care can be personalised for you from an early stage, and have that conversation continue with various professionals involved in your care as the illness progresses. On having had an advance care planning discussion with a social worker, one person commented:

> I've got my life back ... I can't tell you ... it's not what I'd have wanted if you'd given me that magic wand, but it's mine again. I was lost before you know, I didn't know who I was or what was going to happen, it was all such a worry all the time ... but now I know I'm going to stay 'me' for as long as I live, that's precious you know.

We know that uncertainty can be intensely anxiety provoking. While advance care planning cannot help make the future more certain, being able to talk about it can enable individuals to feel more in control as things move forward. For health and social care professionals Deciding Right documentation that captures the heart of these discussions offers a yard stick by which to measure the outcome of the care provided. For family members too, knowing what loved ones want in advance can relieve some of the burden and responsibility from having to make a 'best guess'. As Weinstein (1998) observed, 'bereaved people carry their dead in their consciousness and they live on in memories'. In bereavement, wondering whether they 'got it right' can haunt family members, making their grief more difficult to adjust to. At one of the Deciding Right public engagement events outside a supermarket, one lady approached in visible distress. Her father had died. Surrounded by shoppers she poured out her story of how at the funeral tea, one of her Dad's friends from the pub had come to offer condolences and said how nice the ceremony had been, but that he'd been surprised it was a cremation: her Dad had always said he wanted to be buried. She was devastated. Despite their loving relationship, and all their happy memories together, she still couldn't think about him without an undermining sense that she failed him when he needed her most, and her grief was as real as it had been when he died, twelve years ago. The importance of enabling people to share their concept of a 'good death' with their families, and tell the people that will need to act on those wishes cannot be underestimated. For the lady outside the supermarket, it would have been life changing, 'I didn't know he wanted to be buried, he never told me, I just hope he knows I'm sorry for letting him down' she said. A simple conversation could have avoided twelve years of inner turmoil and helped her to live with the grief over her father's death rather than over her feelings of guilt and failure. Providing people with an opportunity to talk about their future and their wishes can be uncomfortable for professionals, but it can help to alleviate years of ongoing distress for those left behind.

In this era of reduced workforces, increased pressure and dwindling resources, it is acknowledged that proactive advance care planning can be a challenge for social workers and social work departments. However, it is possible that introducing existing clients to their rights and beginning to explore some of their hopes and fears for the future represents a small investment for enormous future gain. Gawande (2014) notes that in one American community, a systematic campaign to get doctors to talk to patients about their end-of-life wishes led to half as many days as the national average spent in hospital in the last six months of life, a reduction in aggressive treatment undertaken, and effective fulfilment of nearly all patients' wishes. This represented a significant reduction in end-of-life care spending, and the same can be true in social care. Georghiou and Bardsley (2014) observe that the proportionate cost per case for people using local authority funded care in the last year of life is significantly higher than other groups. This calculation does not take into account the cost of increasing levels of care often stretching back years, or practitioner time spent responding to crises, managing repeated hospital discharges, and liaising with growing numbers of colleagues. In the American example, discussions of this nature led to more empowered self-aware clients, which enabled practitioners to better anticipate problems, and be more proactive in contingency planning.

Conclusion

The Deciding Right approach promotes more informed and better engaged individuals who are empowered to remain in control of their lives, even into a future where they lose capacity. In turn, this can mean that informal supporters are better equipped, more resilient, and ultimately less reliant on services in a crisis. It goes without saying that this enables smarter use of existing health and social care resources. Advance care planning is not solely social work terrain, nevertheless it is argued that social workers have much to bring to it (APCSW, 2016). Cumbria has found that a change on this scale requires agreement at all levels across the whole social and health care landscape. Working together across professional and organisational boundaries has laid the foundations for 'a better future for the people of Cumbria' (Chaddock, *et al.*, 2014). This has been accomplished through a shared understanding and approach to advance care planning, recording conversations and choices in the standardised documentation, and ensuring that this travels with the person on their journey around the system. By actively seeking to develop a culture of talking about the future, the Deciding Right project in Cumbria is contributing towards an integrated health and social care system that will better meet the needs of those accessing services. This kind of partnership, collaborating to act on a shared understanding and purpose, has been found to work well. In an era of austerity which necessitates creative and innovative approaches, incorporating advance care planning discussions into the core social work task makes economic sense, as well as improving outcomes for individuals at end-of-life. Social workers have access to people at an early stage of their difficulties and are equipped with the skills required to adeptly introduce the subject. In a society reluctant to address end-of-life issues, health and social work professionals pulling together sharing ethos and approach can effectively support individuals to define and realise their end-of-life wishes.

Disclosure statement

No potential conflict of interest was reported by the author.

References

APCSW. (2016) *The Role of Social Work in Palliative, End of Life, and Bereavement Care.* Available from: http://www.apcsw.org.uk/resources

Barclay, S. & Forrest, S. (2007) 'Palliative care: a task for everyone', *British Journal of General Practice*, vol. 57, no. 539, p. 503.

Care Act. (2014) *Elizabeth II*, The Stationary Office, London.

Chaddock, B., Bradley, C. & Laycock, M. (2014) *Implementing Deciding Right in Cumbria.* Available from: http://www.edenvalleyhospice.org/professionals/deciding-right

Department of Health. (2009) *Living Well with Dementia: A National Dementia Strategy*, Department of Health, London.

Detering, KM., Hancock, AD., Reade & Silvester, W. (2010) 'The impact of advance care planning on end of life care in elderly patients: randomised controlled trial', *BMJ*, vol. 340, p. c1345.

Draper, P., Holloway, M. & Adamson, S. (2013) 'A qualitative study of recently bereaved people's beliefs about death: implications for bereavement care', *Journal of Clinical Nursing*, vol. 23 (9–10), pp. 1300–1308.

Gawande, A. (2014) *Being Mortal – Illness, Medicine and What Matters in the End*, Profile Books, London.

Georghiou, T. & Bardsley, M. (2014) *The Cost of Care at the End of Life: Research Report*, Nuffield Trust, London.

Gomes, B. & Higginson, I.J. (2008) 'Where people die (1974–2030): past trends, future projections and implications for care', *Palliative Medicine*, vol. 22, no. 1, pp. 33–41.

Clausen, H., Kendall, M., Murray, S., Worth, A., Boyd, K. & Benton, F. (2005) 'Would palliative care patients benefit from social workers' retaining the traditional 'casework' role rather than working as care managers?', *A Prospective Serial Qualitative Interview Study British Journal Social Work*, vol. 35, no. 2, pp. 277–285.

Hughes, S., Firth, P. & Oliviere, D. (2014) 'Core competencies for palliative care social work in Europe: an EAPC white paper – part 1', *European Journal of Palliative Care*, vol. 21, no. 6, pp. 300–305.

Hughes, S., Firth, P. & Oliviere, D. (2015) 'Core competencies for palliative care social work in Europe: an EAPC white paper – part 2', *European Journal of Palliative Care*, vol. 22, no. 1, pp. 38–44.

Kellehear, A. (2005) *Compassionate Cities: Public Health and End of Life Care*, Routledge, Oxfordshire.

Mental Capacity Act. (2005) *Elizabeth II*, The Stationery Office, London.

National End of Life Care Programme and the College of Social Work. (2012) *The Route to Success in End-of-Life Care – Achieving Quality for Social Work*, TCSW, London.

Northern England Strategic Clinical Networks. (2012) *Deciding right; your life, your choice – a guide to making individual care decisions in advance with children, young people and adults.* Available from: http://www.nescn.nhs.uk/decidingright

Office for National Statistics. (2014) *Deaths Registered in England and Wales 2013–14*, The Stationery Office, London.

Paul, S. (2013) 'Public health approaches to palliative care: the role of the hospice social worker working with children experiencing bereavement,' *British Journal of Social Work*. Available from: www.bjsw.oxfordjournals.org [Accessed 15 Feb 2013].

Prisons and Probation Ombudsman. (2014) *Prisons and Probation Ombudsman Annual Report, 2013–2014*, The Stationery Office, London. Available from: www.ppo.gov.uk [Accessed 21 Jun 2015].

Prince, M., Knapp, M., Guerchet, M., McCrone, P., Prina, M., Comas-Herrera, A., Wittenberg, R., Adelaja, B., Hu, B., King, D., Rehill, A. & Salimkumar, D. (2014) *Dementia UK: Update*, 2nd ed., Alzheimer's Society, London.

Thomas, B. (2012) *Homelessness Kills: an Analysis of the Mortality of Homeless People in Early Twenty-first Century England*, Crisis, London.

Weinstein, J. (1998) '"A proper haunting": the need in mourning to maintain a continuing relationship with the dead', *Journal of Social Work Practice*, vol. 12, no. 1, pp. 93–102.

Yalom, I.S. (2008) *Staring into the Sun: Overcoming the Terror of Death*, Piatkus, London.

Sally Paul [ID]

WORKING WITH COMMUNITIES TO DEVELOP RESILIENCE IN END OF LIFE AND BEREAVEMENT CARE: HOSPICES, SCHOOLS AND HEALTH PROMOTING PALLIATIVE CARE

This paper discusses research undertaken to explore and develop practice between a hospice and two primary schools. Action research was used to increase understanding about current practice in, and with, schools and to explore, implement and evaluate models of practice. Seven practice innovations were identified that are in various stages of being piloted. These innovations can be understood as health promoting palliative care activities, due to the process through which they were designed and their focus on developing the capacity of communities to respond to death, dying and bereavement. They demonstrate the diverse role that hospices, can play in developing how communities experience death, dying and bereavement and propose that a broader lens is employed to understand and facilitate end of life and bereavement services.

Introduction

These are challenging times for palliative care services. Current service provision will not meet the needs of an aging population and this demands consideration about how care and support can best be delivered. Adopting public health approaches to end-of-life care, specifically health promoting palliative care, offers opportunities to address this challenge. It seeks to improve existing services alongside wider social reform that develops death and bereavement friendly communities (Rumbold, 2011). An action research study was undertaken in my role as a hospice social worker to explore and advance education and support around death, dying and bereavement in school communities. This paper begins by discussing the context for this research, exploring how my profession and current practice shaped it. I outline how this experience links to public health approaches to palliative care, focusing on health promoting palliative care and its relevance for both hospice and school communities. I go on to discuss action research as a tool for developing practice, describing the practice innovations that arose as a result of this research. I finish by discussing the practice innovations in relation to health promoting palliative care and the potential role that hospices can play in developing the resilience of school communities to support death, dying and bereavement experiences. Because my research was located in Scotland I have drawn primarily on Scottish legislation and policy, however, my discussion on the role of hospices and health promoting palliative care is inevitably broader than Scotland.

Background

In 2007 I began working as a social worker in a hospice. The Hospice with whom I was employed provides specialist palliative care to a catchment area of almost a third of a million people across a rural area of Scotland. Palliative care is

> an approach that improves the quality of life of patients (adults and children) and their families who are facing problems associated with life-threatening illness [...] This includes addressing practical needs and providing bereavement counselling. It offers a support system to help patients live as actively as possible until death (WHO, 2015).

Specialist palliative care thus involves working with individuals and families both during and after the illness.

My initial role was a newly created position that involved coordinating the organisation's plans for setting up a children's bereavement service, as well as completing other social work tasks within the setting. It was an exciting opportunity, and my senior and I spent a great deal of time liaising with the local community and service providers to design and facilitate the service. Referrals were much greater than anticipated and, six months after I started, we were already holding bereavement groups for children and their parent/carers two (sometimes three) nights per week. Three years into my post, the Hospice management team invited staff to put forward potential research ideas. The children's service was beginning to build reputation for its work in the community and we were receiving increasing numbers of referrals from other professionals as well as requests from schools and social work agencies to provide bereavement training. I had run over 20 groups and, although each group involved different challenges, I was keen to develop my skills and knowledge further. My experience of working with children meant I was becoming increasingly aware of an apparent taboo surrounding death, dying and bereavement, which often resulted in children being excluded from important conversations about significant aspects of their lives. There were some occasions when children were referred for specialist bereavement support unnecessarily. This was due to reticence of the adults to communicate with the child about bereavement issues, referring them on to us when sometimes they had not even asked the child how they were feeling. Broad and Fletcher (1993) argue that the right time for practitioner research is when an experienced professional is ready for a new challenge that involves reflecting on their work and moving forward to find out more. I recognised the significance of providing a bereavement service. I was keen, however, to engage with the social work task from a proactive standpoint, seeking to prevent negative bereavement experiences by developing capacity within children's existing communities to manage death, dying and bereavement. I felt this focus would result in a more positive experience for children, whereby their experiences of death and bereavement were normalised, not pathologised, acknowledged and supported by people with whom existing relationships exist.

My experiences of the children's bereavement service happened alongside policy movements in the UK, which called for discourse and education around death, dying and bereavement to be promoted (Department of Health, 2008, 2010; Scottish Government, 2008). Since the introduction of these policies, a variety of advances have since been made that focus on creating more openness around death, dying and bereavement. In 2009, in England and Wales, 'Dying Matters', a national coalition to promote greater public awareness and discussion of issues relating to death, dying and bereavement was developed. This included the introduction of a 'Dying Matters' awareness week, which has been identified as providing end-of-life care services with a defined opportunity to open up discourse on death, dying and bereavement (Paul and Sallnow, 2013). In Scotland, a short-life working group was set up, specifically addressing palliative and end-of-life care from a public health and health promotion perspective to facilitate a wider discussion of death, dying and bereavement across society. In 2011, this led to the establishment of the 'Good Life, Good Death, Good Grief Alliance', which seeks to provide a network and resources to raise public awareness and promote community involvement in death, dying and bereavement (goodlifedeathgrief 2012). This was further emphasised by the Scottish Government in their *Strategic Framework for Action on Palliative Care (2015)*, which highlights the need to establish 'greater openness about death, dying and bereavement' and recognise 'the wider sources of support within communities that enable people to live and die well'. These developments go beyond developing discourse around death, dying and bereavement to involving the community in addressing end-of-life and bereavement care issues. Such approaches are recognised in a report by DEMOS, a British cross-party think-tank, which asks for a '"Big Society" response to a dying population in which civic, mutual and self-help solutions play a much greater role' (Leadbeater and Garber, 2010, p. 16). From this perspective, end-of-life and bereavement care is everyone's responsibility, thus situating palliative care as a public health issue and identifying associated approaches as an effective way to improve and develop care.

Public health approaches to palliative care: health promoting palliative care

Issues related to death, dying and bereavement have previously been excluded from public health discourse. Public health activities have historically been referred to as life-affirming, avoiding death and dying by focusing on preventing and controlling illness, disease, injury and premature death (Kellehear and Young, 2007; Lupton,

1995). Combining public health approaches with palliative care is, however, now recognised as offering a powerful way to achieve meaningful end-of-life care for the majority of people (Conway, 2007; Kellehear, 1999a; Stjernswärd *et al.*, 2007). This involves moving focus from traditional public health models, which concentrate on the cure and treatment of disease, to 'new' public health models that focus on equity of care 'and on attempting to break down barriers between professional groups and lay people' (Cohen and Deliens, p. 11). From a 'new' public health perspective, public health approaches to palliative care thus involve working to promote openness and challenge stigmas related to death, dying and bereavement as well as empowering communities to draw on their own resources and community supports to adapt and cope. These principles are equally essential to the role and task of social work and I have argued elsewhere the relevance of a public health approach to palliative care for the social work profession (Paul, 2013).

Health promotion is a central feature of the 'new' public health. It recognises health as a multidimensional concept involving physical, social and emotional aspects and is a concept 'premised on the understanding that the behaviours in which we engage and the circumstances in which we live impact on our health, and that appropriate changes will improve health' (Bennett and Murphy, 1997, p. 7). In 1986, the World Health Organisation (WHO) produced the Ottawa Charter for Health Promotion. Five strategies were identified to support and maintain health that included building public health policy, creating supportive environments, strengthening community actions, developing personal skills and reorienting health services (WHO, 1986, p. 2). In 1999, Allan Kellehear explicitly applied the WHO principles of health promotion to palliative care (Kellehear, 1999b). The notion of health promoting palliative care thus emerged, broadening out the remit of palliative care providers from the personal, i.e. supporting individual families, to the community. According to Street (2007), palliative care from a health promotion perspective is

> not only directed at the care of individuals [...] but is also concerned with the social and community environment [and] public policies and community services [which] enable communities to cope with the inevitability of death and consciously support loss, grief, dying and bereavement, especially in the most vulnerable community members (p. 105).

Health promoting palliative care is thus a holistic approach that recognises and builds on existing strengths and skills within the wider community. Although it is only one public health approach, health promotion is usable in small settings (Kellehear, 2005). This affirms that end-of-life care providers are in a position to initiate and/ or provide leadership in health promotion activities through developing community partnerships, which aim to establish sustainable activities addressing issues surrounding death, dying and bereavement (Kellehear and O'Connor, 2008; Street, 2007).

A survey of UK palliative care services found that public health approaches to palliative care was a priority for the majority of services (Paul and Sallnow, 2013). A review of 28 projects in England further revealed interest and commitment to the field (Barry and Patel, 2013). In Scotland, schools have been identified as an important target for health promoting palliative care to ensure that children develop the skills and capacity to talk about, and cope with, death, dying and bereavement

(Scottish Government, 2010). Moreover, schools have been identified as key in supporting and responding to children's bereavement experiences (Hemmings, 1995; Rowling, 2003). In the afore mentioned survey of UK palliative care services, working with schools was the most common type of work done in the community, identified by 73% of respondents (Paul and Sallnow, 2013). This suggests that working with schools is on the agenda of palliative care services and is deemed to be something worthwhile. There is, however, a lack of literature sharing this work and discussing the extent to which such activities are health promoting. Moreover, the practice of introducing health promoting palliative care occurs largely within clinical healthcare settings (Kellehear, 2005). This indicates that health promoting palliative care activities are often defined by the boundaries of an institution/organisation as opposed to working with communities more broadly. It has been argued that a reason for this limited perspective is that palliative care organisations lack time, funding and training/understanding of health promotion activities (Kellehear, 2005; Rosenberg and Yates, 2010). This analysis corresponds with my knowledge and awareness of current UK projects, specifically those working with children, which use the hospice as a 'specialist' site from which to facilitate activities for the community (Hartley, 2009; Turner, 2010). Although these projects are undoubtedly worthwhile they still situate palliative care professionals as central to the activity.

Kellehear (2005, p. 156) offers a 'Big Seven Checklist' as a guide to understanding 'genuine' health promoting palliative care activities. The seven questions are:

(1) In what way does the project help prevent social difficulties around death, dying, loss or care?
(2) In what way do they harm-minimise difficulties we may not be able to prevent around death, dying, loss or care?
(3) In what ways can these activities be understood as early interventions along the journey of death, dying, loss or care?
(4) In what ways do these activities alter/change a setting or environment for the better in terms of our present or future responses to death, dying, loss or care?
(5) In what way are the proposed activities participatory – borne, partnered and nurtured by community member?
(6) How sustainable will the activities or programmes be without your future input?
(7) How can we evaluate their success of usefulness so that we can justify their presence, their funding and their ongoing support?

The checklist highlights community ownership, collaboration and participation as essential to a health promoting approach to palliative care. This draws attention to the importance of working *with* communities, to engage them in a process of identifying and addressing end-of-life and bereavement care issues that are pertinent to their own specific needs, i.e. transferring power rather than maintaining it. The check-list also identifies the importance of developing activities that are based on early intervention and harm-reduction that involves normalising death, dying and bereavement and proactively preparing individuals and communities for related experiences. Nevertheless, there is little research that has used this checklist to help understand and define activities ran by palliative care services. In planning my study

I identified a need for more research that explores and develops activities initiated by hospices, specifically those with schools, using the checklist to critique the extent to which such activities confirm the fundamental principles of true health promoting palliative care.

Action research: a research approach to practice development

I have confirmed that engaging with the social work task to advance practice was important to me. It was also important to my organisation, which was keen to see specific practice innovations developed as a result of funding the research. This prompted me to choose an action research methodology which aims to both increase knowledge, experience and understanding of a current situation and engage in a process of change (Coghlan and Brannick, 2001; Creswell, 2007; Winter and Munn-Giddings, 2001). It is operational field research that deals with everyday issues of practice to increase effectiveness (McKernan, 1996) and involves a spiral of steps composed of planning, action and evaluation/critical reflection of the action in order to plan subsequent events. It sits within participatory research paradigm that involves connecting people, subjects, objects and their environments (Hockley and Froggatt, 2006). It is a developmental process in which participants resolve the issues in question. Theory in action research thus attempts to 'bridge theory and practice but also generate new ways of understanding practice' (Noffke in Noffke and Somekh, 2009, p. 10).

The research was undertaken in two primary schools in Scotland, starting in August 2011. Schools were invited to take part due to their proximity to the Hospice, size and denomination; one non-denominational school (NDS) and one Roman Catholic school (RCS) were selected to see if this impacted on developed practice (in Scotland 14% of all schools are denominational, the bulk of which are Roman Catholic). Participants included anyone who might be involved in potential practice innovations, including hospice and school staff, children and parents/carers. Potential adult participants were given verbal and written information about the research and invited to self-select as research participants. For children, a letter was sent home informing parent/carers that the research was happening in the school and that the researcher would be inviting their child to participate. They were then asked to opt their child out if they wished. For those children who were not opted out, the researcher provided written and verbal information about the research. The children were later asked to fill in a brief form indicating their interest in partici-pating and/or if they had any questions. As a result of this process, 22 participants were recruited from the Hospice, 32 participants (seven staff, 21 children and four parents) were recruited at RSC and 18 participants (six staff and 12 children) were recruited at NDS. No parents/carers agreed to participate in the research at NDS. Informed consent was sought from all participants. Owing to the duration of the action research, consent was kept a live issue so that participants were aware they could withdraw from the research at any time. Ethical review procedures were completed and approved at The University of Edinburgh, the Hospice and Local Authority (LA) in which the schools and research was based.

Phase 1 (preparation and scoping):

A literature review, visits to other hospices and four focus groups with Hospice staff to determine the extent to which they already engaged with primary schools, the focus of this work and areas for development.

Phase 2 (exploration):

A series of interviews and focus groups with children, parent and school staff participants toexplore current practice in relation to death, dying and bereavement and engage in a process of change.

Phase 3 (planning and developing model(s) for practice):

Dissemination of written reports based on the findings generated in phases one and two and meetings with key stakeholders to discuss, identify and develop possible practice developments.

Phase 4 (pilot developed practice):

Pilot of the identified and developed practice innovations across hospice and/or school settings.

Phase 5 (evaluate developed practice):

Evaluation of practice innovations in partnership with key stakeholders. Practice is adapted and developed asper evaluation findings.

FIGURE 1 Overview of research phases.

The action research was conducted over five phases. Figure 1 describes the detail of these phases. The interviews and focus groups in phase 2 were piloted prior to this and were facilitated using an interview and focus group guide. The interviews and focus groups each lasted approximately forty minutes to fit in with the school timetable. They were digitally recorded and then transcribed. Data from these initial phases was analysed thematically with themes derived from the data.

This paper reports on the research undertaken in Phases 1, 2 and 3. The findings from Phases 4 and 5 are on-going and will be reported elsewhere.

Findings from phase three: the identified practice innovations

Both research sites identified three practice innovations to take forward. An additional practice idea was also identified by the LA Education Services, as a result of the action research process at one of the schools. The activities are summarised in Table 1, which, for ease of discussion, have been numbered from one to seven.

I have discussed elsewhere the main themes deriving from these innovations and what this suggests for the role of Hospices working with schools (forthcoming). Given the scale of this research, and the methodology used, it is hard to draw general conclusions concerning the role of Hospices working with school communities beyond this context. The innovations are site specific and as a result only describe the role of the Hospice working with *that* particular school.

Regardless there are some interesting characteristics of the innovations worthy of further examination. First, it is apparent that the majority of these practice innovations involve mobilising those already caring for, and interacting with, children to be actively involved in providing support and education around death, dying and bereavement. Second, not all the innovations focus on improving services run by the Hospice. Practice developments (3) and (4) involved improving current services ran by the Hospice, yet, the remaining practice innovations were concerned with transforming practice in school communities to better cope with death, dying and bereavement. Third, the focus of all the activities directly relate to the principles of health promoting palliative care and suggests that Hospices do play a key role in developing related activities.

To assess the extent of this role, I have explored how these practice developments address Kellehear's (2005) 'Big Seven Checklist' for health promoting palliative care activities, as identified in the literature and demonstrated through the research experience.

Practice innovations and the 'Big Seven Checklist'

Table 2 outlines the 'Big Seven Checklist', detailing how I consider each practice development to meet the specified criteria. With the exception of practice development (6), provide parent/carer workshops, all of the practice developments are in line with the checklist. This suggests they can be viewed as genuine health promoting palliative care activities. There are a number of gaps under practice development (6), primarily because during phase three it was intended that this activity would be discussed with parents/carers at NDS and a subsequent plan for advancing this activity produced. However, to date this discussion has not taken place and it is unknown if and how it might progress.

I have asserted that the majority of the developments meet all of the first three questions on the check-list due to their focus on establishing death and bereavement as a normal human experience, seeking to develop individual and community capacity to cope with such experiences. Practice developments (3) and (4) (use fundraising to raise awareness of hospice care), however, can only be understood as an early intervention due to their focus on informing as opposed to empowering.

TABLE 1 Summary of practice developments

	Practice development	Description
RCS	(1) Integrate health and death education throughout the curriculum	Create and implement an education programme that integrates education on health, illness, death and bereavement into the curriculum across all ages. To be led by school staff with some input from Hospice staff where needed
	(2) Provide bereavement training for school staff	School and Hospice staff to jointly develop and design a bereavement training programme that provides information on childhood bereavement and the skills to manage related issues, where appropriate, in the school setting. The training will be facilitated by Hospice staff and aimed at all school staff, including teachers and support staff
	(3) Provide information about the Hospice during the Hospice 'Go Yellow' fundraising event	Children and Hospice staff to jointly develop materials to use with the Hospice 'Go Yellow' annual schools fundraising event. The materials should inform school staff and pupils about the role of the Hospice in the community and how money raised is spent
NDS	(4) Carry out activities about the Hospice during the Hospice 'Schoolfriends' fundraising event	Children and school staff to jointly develop a series of activities for school children about the role of the Hospice that can be carried out when participating in the Hospice 'Schoolfriends' fundraising event
	(5) Provide bereavement training for school staff	School and Hospice staff to adapt the bereavement training programme designed with RCS (practice development two) to suit the needs of NDS. Facilitated by Hospice staff with all school staff
	(6) Provide a parent/carer bereavement workshop	School staff to establish need for a parent/carer workshop on the bereavement needs of children and the role of the Hospice in the community. Hospice staff to develop and facilitate workshop
LA education services	(7) Develop a bereavement policy	School staff, Hospice staff and children to develop a LA schools bereavement policy. The policy should include specific guidelines on how to respond to bereavement in school communities

Informing and educating are key features of all the innovations. This includes education that raises awareness of end-of-life and bereavement issues as well as developing capacity to support related experiences. For example, practice development (1) (curriculum development), relates to what Rowling (2003) deems as external agencies having a preventative role with school communities. This includes activities designed to educate and support children so that they are better able to cope with loss and change. Practice development (7) (policy development), includes informing schools communities on the impact of bereavement on children and their responsibility to ensure that procedures are in place to support such experiences.

TABLE 2 The practice developments and Kellehear's (2005) 'Big Seven Checklist'

'Big Seven Checklist'	Practice developments				
	(1) Death and health education in the curriculum	(2) (5) Bereavement training to school staff	(3) (4) Fundraising to raise awareness	(6) Parent/carer workshops	(7) Bereavement policy
In what way does/can the project					
(1) Help prevent social difficulties around death, dying and loss? or (2) Harm-minimize difficulties we may not be able to prevent around death, dying, loss or care? or (3) Be understood as early interventions along the journey of death, dying, loss or care?	• Health and death education is part of the syllabus (1,2,3) • Open culture of talking about death and loss (1) • Children aware of issues related to death and grief before they happen (2,3)	• Develop skills and confidence of school staff to address bereavement (1,2,3) • Develops culture on supporting bereaved children in school (1) • Raises awareness of bereavement needs of children (2) • Raises awareness of specialist support to be accessed when needed (2)	• Introduces hospice care to school communities (3) • Uses accessible, child friendly language (3)	• Develop skill and confidence of parents/carers to notice and address bereavement (1,2,3) • Raises awareness of bereavement needs of children (2) • Raises awareness of specialist support to be accessed when needed (2)	• Establishes culture of supporting bereaved children in school (1) • Raises awareness of bereavement needs of children and provides guidance on how to meet these needs (2,3)
(4) In what ways do these activities *alter/change a setting or environment for the better* in terms of our present or future responses to death, dying, loss or care?	Establishes death as a normal part of life. Develops skills to manage loss and change	Assists in creating a responsive and supportive bereavement culture in school	Assists in breaking down stigma of hospice care	Assists in creating a responsive and supportive bereavement culture in school and at home	Establishes a supportive bereavement culture in all schools in the LA
(5) In what way are the proposed activities *participatory – borne*, partnered and nurtured by community member?	Action research	Action research	Action research	Action research	Action research
(6) How *sustainable* will the activities or programmes be without your future input?	Rolling programme in school	Led by Hospice DEPDR. Ongoing training needs identified by school	Led by Hospice fundraising team	Action research	Ongoing policy, implemented across all schools
(7) How can we *evaluate* their success of usefulness so that we can justify their presence, their funding and their ongoing support?	School audit and evaluation procedures	Led by Hospice DEPDR	Led by Hospice fundraising team	Action research	School audit and evaluation procedures

Education on death, dying and bereavement experiences has been highlighted as a method of harm reduction as it is associated with a number of benefits that relate to emotional wellbeing. For example, education on death and dying has been identified as enabling and preparing people to manage individual experiences of, and support those impacted by, death and loss (Kellehear and O'Connor, 2008). It has also been asserted as equipping people with the tools and language to address difficult aspects of loss and death (Jackson and Colwell, 2001; McGovern and Barry, 2000) and providing people with an opportunity to clarify values, meanings and attitudes towards death (Feifel, 1977). Providing information and education on end-of-life and bereavement care has been a key feature of the hospice movement since it was first established (Hockley, 1997). These innovations suggest however that education is provided by Hospice staff where needed (such as via fundraising and bereavement training) but is also designed and delivered by school communities.

In relation to question four (alter an environment for the better), it is not possible to tell how the practice developments will change the school environment until they are fully evaluated. Nonetheless, by considering the purpose of the activities, it can be assumed that their main intention is to either raise awareness of end-of-life care issues or improve how schools respond to loss and bereavement, both of which aim to positively affect school communities. This question, however, highlights a key criticism of health promoting activities. Pomerleau and McKee (2005) assert that such activities assume 'that it is justifiable to constrain the freedom of one individual to benefit the population as a whole' (p. 10). Health promotion is therefore not value free and systemically changing an environment, for example by policy and curriculum development, prioritises one value over another. This demonstrates the significance of question five, that all activities are participatory borne, but also suggests that there is value in the Hospice developing activities that are local and relevant to specific community groups rather than more broadly.

Initially, question five (participatory borne activities) seemed an easy question to fulfil given that the developments were a result of action research which focuses on developing practice which is shaped and owned by communities members. Yet, although research participants identified all of the activities, parents/carers were not involved in choosing practice development (6) (parent/carer workshop). Instead, this development was identified by school staff whom argued that it would be a beneficial practice development for parents/carers. As no parents/carers were involved in this decision this practice development was therefore not genuinely participatory borne and does not meet the guidelines for health promoting palliative care. This identifies power within communities that can influence how practice is shaped by determining and responding to need without actually involving the people whom the practice is aimed at. It highlights that in designing and responding to end-of-life care and bereavement issues the Hospice must consider whose views are included and whose are not to ensure that practice is relevant.

It can be argued that all of the activities are sustainable, therefore meeting question six, as it is planned that all of the developments will continue without my on-going involvement. Nevertheless, at the time of writing it is not possible to say if this is the case as the majority of activities are still in the process of being piloted. Moreover, it is planned that the activities will be continued by those best placed to do so, meaning that I will not be in the position of an external facilitator to maintain the momentum of the work. Instead they rely on motivation, and time available, of the responsible staff. This is potentially in keeping with the multi-disciplinary, focus of health promotion, which places emphasis on cooperative relationships and involves action from all involved parties (Peterson and Lupton, 1996). This draws attention to the importance of working *with* communities, to engage them in a process of identifying and addressing end-of-life care issues pertinent to their own specific needs, i.e. transferring power rather than maintaining it. However, a possible challenge in initiating activities that seek to empower communities to develop and carry out activities is then the extent to which such activities can be supported and monitored. Practice developments (1) (curriculum development) and (7) (policy development), will be incorporated into existing school frameworks and because of this is it likely that these two developments will be sustainable. This, however, is not a feature of all activities. If focus continues to be placed on developing health promoting palliative care activities it is important therefore that systems and procedures are in place for acknowledging, reviewing and sharing these activities.

Question seven (evaluate success) was difficult to answer as the practice developments are led by different groups of people and the level to which these groups prioritise evaluation is unknown. It is likely that practice developments (1) (curriculum development), (2) and (5) (bereavement training) and (7) (policy development) will be evaluated because they have pre-existing evaluation procedures. Yet, evaluating their success or usefulness is not necessarily included within these procedures. For example, the Hospice Department of Education, Practice Development and Research (DEPDR) always evaluate participant experience after any training programme, yet it does not always evaluate if and how the training has been put into action. Lupton (1995) criticises health promoting activities for often being short term and below the threshold to make sustainable effects. This suggests that, when developing health promoting palliative care activities, focus should be placed on the purpose and method of evaluation from the beginning so that this can be incorporated effectively, including measuring the impact of such activities.

Conclusion

This research set out to explore practice between a Hospice and two primary schools that advanced education and support around death, dying and bereavement experiences. It was a product of my practice experience as a hospice social worker coupled with an awareness and interest in the emerging field of public health approaches to palliative care, specifically health promoting palliative care. The research did not set out specifically to create health promoting palliative care activities: such practice and its significance to end-of-life and bereavement care was discussed as a basis from which to explore and critique practice developments arising from the research process. Yet, the majority of practice innovations that arose as a result of this research were not based on the Hospice delivering specific services to schools but mobilising those involved in caring for children to be actively involved in providing support and education around death, dying and bereavement. By discussing these innovations alongside the principles of health promoting palliative, community ownership, participation and capacity building were highlighted. This, in turn, identified the significance of designing activities around the needs of school communities, which are led, but not owned by, palliative care professionals. I have argued therefore that the practice innovations can be understood as health promoting palliative care activities due to their focus on developing the resilience of school communities to cope and manage issues relating to death, dying and bereavement experiences. Furthermore, I have suggested that hospices are well placed to engage with and develop health promoting activities. With this focus, school communities are viewed by hospices as an equal partner in providing quality care and education around death, dying and bereavement for children and integral to providing meaningful support. Engaging with the social work task from a proactive standpoint was a key focus of this research. The identified activities engage proactively with death, dying and bereavement by concentrating on developing the education and skills of children, and those around them, to cope with experiences related to death, dying and bereavement. This highlights the relevance of public health approaches to palliative care for social workers and the important role that social work professionals have in developing practice in this area.

Acknowledgements

The author would like to thank Professor Viviene Cree and Professor Scott Murray for their research supervision and Professor Heather Richardson for her helpful comments on earlier versions of this paper. The author would also like to thank Strathcarron Hospice for funding and supporting the PhD research.

Disclosure statement

No potential conflict of interest was reported by the author.

ORCID

Sally Paul ⓘ http://orcid.org/0000-0003-1690-8411

References

Barry, V., & Patel, M. (2013) *An Overview of Compassionate Communities in England*, Murray Hall Community Trust and National Council for Palliative Care Dying Matters, London.
Bennett, P. & Murphy, S. (1997) *Psychology and Health Promotion*, Open University Press, Buckingham.
Broad, B. & Fletcher, C. (1993) *Practitioner Social Work Research in Action*, Whiting & Birch, London.

Coghlan, D. & Brannick, T. (2001) *Doing Action Research in Your Own Organization*, Sage, London.

Conway, S. (2007) 'The changing face of death: implications for public health', *Critical Public Health*, vol. 17, no. 3, pp. 195–202.

Creswell, J. W. (2007) *Qualitative Inquiry and Research Design: Choosing Among Five Approaches*, 2nd ed., Sage, Thousand Oaks, CA.

Department of Health. (2008) *End of Life Care Strategy – Promoting High Quality Care for Adults at the End of Life*, Department of Health, London.

Department of Health, S. S. a. P. S. (2010) *Living Matters, Dying Matters: A Palliative and End of Life Care Strategy for Adults in Northern Ireland*, Department of Health, Social Services and Public Safety, Belfast.

Feifel, H. (1977) 'Death and dying in modern America', *Death Education*, vol. 6, pp. 69–174.

Goodlifedeathgrief. (2012) www.goodlifedeathgrief.org.uk [Last Accessed 17th March 2012].

Hartley, N. (2009) 'Creating healthier attitudes to death and dying', *Hospice Information Bulletin, Help the Hospices*, vol. 6, no. 4, p. 1.

Hemmings, P. (1995) 'Social work intervention with bereaved children', *Journal of Social Work Practice*, vol. 9, no. 2, pp. 109–130.

Hockley, J. (1997) 'The evolution of the hospice approach', in *New Themes in Palliative Care*, eds D. Clark, J. Hockley & S. Ahmedzai, Open Univeristy Press, Buckingham.

Hockley, J. & Froggatt, K. (2006) 'The development of palliative care knowledge in care homes for older people: the place of action research', *Palliative Medicine*, vol. 20, no. 8, pp. 835–843.

Jackson, M. & Colwell, J. (2001) 'Talking to children about death', *Mortality*, vol. 6, no. 3, pp. 321–325.

Kellehear, A. (1999) *Health-promoting Palliative Care*, Oxford University Press, Melbourne.

Kellehear, A. (1999) 'Health-promoting palliative care: developing a social model for practice', *Mortality*, vol. 4, no. 1, pp. 75–82.

Kellehear, A. (2005) *Compassionate cities: public health and end-of-life care*, Routledge, London.

Kellehear, A. & O'Connor, D. (2008) 'Health-promoting palliative care: a practice example', *Critical Public Health*, vol. 18, no. 1, pp. 111–115.

Kellehear, A. & Young, B. (2007) 'Resilient communities', in *Resilience in Palliative Care*, eds B. Monroe & D. Oliviere, Oxford University Press, Oxford.

Leadbeater, C. & Garber, J. (2010) *Dying for Change*, DEMOS, London.

Lupton, D. (1995) *The Imperative of Health: Public Health and the Regulated Body*, London: Sage.

McGovern, M. & Barry, M. (2000) 'Death education: knowledge, attitudes and perspectives of Irish parents and teachers', *Death Studies*, vol. 24, pp. 325–333.

McKernan, J. (1996) *Curriculumn Action Research: A Handbook of Methods and Resources for the Reflective Practitioner*, 2nd ed., Kogan Page, London.

Noffke, S.E. & Somekh, B. (2009) *The SAGE Handbook of Educational Action Research*, Sage, Los Angeles, CA.

Paul, S. (2013) 'Public Health Approaches to Palliative Care: The Role of the Hospice Social Worker Working with Children Experiencing Bereavement', *British Journal of Social Work*, vol. 43, no. 2, pp. 249–263.

Paul, S., & Sallnow, L. (2013) 'Public health approaches to end of life care in the UK: an online survey of palliative care services', *British Medical Journal: Supportive and Palliative Care*, vol. 3, no. 2, pp. 196–199.

Peterson, A.R. & Lupton, D. (1996) *The New Public Health: Health and Self in the Age of Risk*, Sage, London.

Pomerleau, J. & McKee, M. (2005) *Issues in Public Health*, Open University Press, Maidenhead.

Rosenberg, J. P. & Yates, P. M. (2010) 'Health promotion in palliative care: the case for conceptual congruence', *Critical Public Health*, vol. 20, no. 2, pp. 201–210.

Rowling, L. (2003) *Grief in School Communities: Effective Support Strategies*, Open University Press, Buckingham.

Rumbold, B. (2011) 'Health promoting palliative care and dying in old age', in *Living with Aging and Dying: Palliative and End of Life Care for Older People*, eds M. Gott & C. Ingelton, Oxford University Press, Oxford.

Scottish Government. (2008) *Living and Dying Well: A National Action Plan for Palliative and End of Life Care in Scotland, Edited by Scotland. H.*, The Scottish Government, Edinburgh.

Scottish Government. (2010) *Short Life Working Group 7: Final Report. Addressing Palliative and End of Life Care from a Public Health and Health Promotion Perspective: Facilitating Wider Discussion of Death, Dying and Bereavement across Society*. Scottish Government, Edinburgh.

Scottish Government. (2015) *Strategic Framework for Action on Palliative Care*, Scottish Government, Edinburgh

Stjernswärd, J., Foley, K. M. & Ferris, F. D. (2007) 'The public health strategy for palliative care', *Journal of Pain and Symptom Management*, vol. 33, no. 5, pp. 486–493.

Street, A. (2007) 'Leading the way: innovative health-promoting palliative care', *Contemporary Nurse*, vol. 27, pp. 104–106.

WHO (1986) Ottawa Charter for Health Promotion, Ottawa: World Health Organisation.

WHO. (2015) *Fact Sheet on Palliative Care*, Fact sheet N°402, July 2015.

Winter, R. & Munn-Giddings, C. (2001) *A Handbook for Action Research in Health and Social Care*, Routledge, London.

Jason Davidson

DOES THE CULTURE OF MODERN DAY PALLIATIVE CARE SOCIAL WORK LEAVE ROOM FOR LEADERSHIP?

This paper describes research undertaken as part of an MA study in leadership. It draws on interviews with six high profile leaders at the fore front of end of life care sector in the UK. Its findings and emerging themes offer insights about the opportunities for social work leaders in palliative care in the future and how the profession and palliative care sector address current barriers to taking advantage of such opportunity. The main focus of this paper is leadership related to palliative care social work. However, it relates to much broader themes including the history, politics and culture of this profession and the requirements for leadership on the part of social work in the broader contexts of health and social care.

Leadership in palliative care social work: a personal and professional journey

Social workers have made a significant contribution to end of life care in the UK for decades. However, as a social worker practicing in palliative care today I find myself constrained by the lack of social work role models in a position of leadership. Without a leadership role model to whom and what do I aspire? Where can I go to explore strategic issues relevant to my work from a social work perspective?

This appears to be a loneliness that is specific to social work in the broader context of palliative care. In contrast, many colleagues in nursing and medicine working in the specialty appear to embrace a concept of leadership in their work and aspire to develop this aspect of their role. They are supported in this journey, as they enjoy well-worn career pathways to more senior positions.

In 2009 I took up my first hospice social work post. I was excited, passionate and ambitious. Anticipating a new career for the future, I wondered very early on what pathways were available to someone like me and where might they lead.

It quickly became obvious that there was no blueprint for the journey that I wanted to pursue towards a leadership role. I recall a salutary conversation with the chief executive of the organisation for which I worked at that time. We were on our way to a local NHS conference on strategy and end of life care. Halfway through the journey he turned to me and said 'I didn't think social workers were interested in strategy'. My bubble was burst. If he, as a seasoned leader couldn't see the potential contribution of social workers to high level leadership then I realised I had a long way to go.

In addition I soon began to realise that this ambition was not one that was always shared widely by my professional colleagues. In my view, in the context of palliative care, we are a profession that often shies away from the limelight.

The late Dame Cicely Saunders founder of the modern hospice movement who was herself a social worker managed to become arguably the most significant leader in palliative care. So, if my experience is anything to go by, why does a group of highly skilled professionals find itself feeling fearful about their future and increasingly worried about their value within a hierarchy of professionals working in end of life care – an area of work that remains topical and high on many people's agenda?

Drawing on my own experience and anecdotal evidence I believe there to be real challenges around provision of high quality end of life care in the UK; additionally there are significant risks related to the future of palliative care social work in the UK. If these challenges and risks are to be addressed, there is an urgent need for leadership of the profession, and strong strategic thinking about its contribution to end of life care in the future, and the shape of such care from a social perspective.

This was the point where my quest for answers began and plans for this study evolved. I was interested to hear the views of existing leaders in the sector and to explore their ideas and how they related to my own. This paper goes onto describe that research in more detail, revealing important themes that are pertinent to the development of social work as a profession today and in the future.

Background

End of life care needs improvement

Health and social care services across the UK need to do more to improve end of life care. Recent research shows that a significant amount of those people who are dying in the UK are not receiving the right support and care. The charity Marie Curie and the London School of Economics in their report *Equity in the provision of palliative and end of life care in the UK* (April 2015) who reported on the experience of carers, suggest seven out of every ten people with a terminal illness in the UK don't receive the care and support they need. These inequities must be removed from the system. Everyone in the UK who is living with a terminal illness deserves to get the right care and support, at the right time and in the right place.

Recent investigations by the parliamentary and health service ombudsman into complaints about end of life care highlights significant failures within the NHS, in providing palliative care. The consequences of these failures for both the dying and those left behind are described in the report in six harrowing case stories. Unfortunately, these are not isolated incidents. In their report *Dying without Dignity* (2015) the parliamentary and health service ombudsman calls for more access to palliative care services and better leadership. Attending to inequalities is arguably a role for social work.

Whilst some improvements have been made in recent years to the end of life care needs of some of our more marginalised groups in the UK such as people who have a learning disability. However, we still have a long way to go. *Death by Indifference* (2007) a report by Mencap about institutional discrimination within the NHS, highlighted how people with a learning disability were receiving poorer healthcare. The report presented the stories of six individuals who Mencap believed died unnecessarily in NHS settings. Unfortunately, five years later Mencap produced a progress report which was titled *Death by Indifference: 74 deaths and counting* (2012) confirming that many of the original reasons for poor quality care still remain.

Efforts to improve end of life care are underway

Current and anticipated changes to the demographic and cultural landscape have ensured that end of life care is afforded increasing central importance in public policy: the fastest growing population group in the UK is people aged over 85 years. Social and health care policy is in a phase of rapid and radical change as it pursues government policy of supporting people to remain in their own homes for as long as they might wish (National End of Life Care Programme, 2010).

Some significant guidance now exists to help hospices and other providers of palliative and end of life care prepare for the future.

In 2008 the Department of Health's End of Life Care Strategy and accompanying implementation programme intended to change the 'culture' and experience of dying in the UK on three different levels: widen society's awareness, service user experience and the professional and service delivery infrastructure. A programme was then set up to devise a framework for social care. One of the key objectives of the framework was to *strengthen the specialism of palliative care social work*. Amongst other things the framework recommended that stakeholders establish a network of social care leads across social care and *promote better links between social and health care and other services* (National End of Life Care Programme, 2010).

In 2010 the think tank Demos published a report entitled *Dying for Change* which highlighted some of the challenges facing hospices in the future (Leadbeater and Garber, 2010). They confirmed that radical change in the way that services are organised and delivered is essential to meet the needs and preferences of the UK population reaching the end of its life in the future. Hospice UK, 2012 (formally Help the Hospices, www.helpthehospices.org.uk/commission), the national umbrella charity responded to this by setting up the Commission into the future of hospice care (2012) to provide guidance, information and options for hospices to inform their strategic position and offerings in the next ten to twenty years. It is notable that there is no specific reference to social work in any of its recommendations regarding the way forward.

Even so, there is guidance provided by the Commission that is pertinent to the role of social workers in end of life care in the future. It identified six key operating principles. The first principle proposed that hospices need to become *a bigger player and a bigger influencer* within the larger health and social care system. The commission suggests that developing stronger and more high profile leadership is essential to achieve this.

In July 2014 the UK saw the end of the Liverpool Care Pathway (LCP). The LCP was an approach to care that included a complex set of interventions and was essentially an attempt to replicate in hospitals the standard of care found in many hospices. An independent review of the pathway was carried out and recommendations were made that dying patients should instead have individualised care plans (Independent Review of the Liverpool Care Pathway, 2014). This was in many respects the start of a concerted effort on the part of Government and others to shift the focus away from pathways to more individualised person centered care.

Social work has an important part to play in improving end of life care

There is currently a major drive in hospice care to implement public health approaches to transform end of life care services. One such approach is that which promotes compassionate communities – in which local communities and their members provide the majority of the care. *A compassionate community gives ordinary people the skills to be able to address the issues raised by the end of life and other losses* (www.nhs.uk). Community engagement is one of the structural foundations of the social work profession and emerging models of care such as this which move away from traditional models of medical care open up a host of opportunities for palliative care social work to demonstrate its unique offerings.

Social workers are leaders in anti-oppressive and anti-discriminatory practice and work hard in palliative care to ensure that people receiving services remain central to decisions about their care. Within their role they will often give attention to inequalities in provision. This role is enacted at multiple levels – national, organisational and for the individual patient. One of the main tasks for the palliative care social worker is to talk openly to patients and their families and carers about death and dying to ensure their needs and preferences are articulated and acknowledged.

Palliative care social workers may struggle to be part of this improvement

In April 2012 the Centre for Workforce Intelligence in their publication 'The future social worker workforce: an analysis of risks and opportunities' (2012) stated that in England there were 87, 442 social workers registered with the GSCC (General Social Care Council). The National Association of Palliative Care Social Workers (APCSW) state on their website that they currently have a membership of over two hundred social workers. Whilst these figures highlight the specialism of palliative care social work, they also highlight their relative scarcity and by implication some vulnerability.

There is some evidence that the work for which they have been renowned, namely emotional support as part of a multi professional team in addressing 'total pain' is also at risk. As social work in the UK has shifted towards the management of risk and a focus on outcomes over process, reports suggest that *therapeutic interventions with dying and bereaved people have come to be seen as a luxury that mainstream social work cannot afford* (NEoLCP, 2012). The report goes on to say that specialist palliative care social workers remain, but *shrinking numbers and redefined roles and functions have led to feelings that their specialism is under threat* (NEoLCP, 2012).

Regardless, the literature confirms a vital role for social workers at practice and policy levels, supporting individualised care, and that which addresses social needs through community action alongside any professional interventions. What is less clear from the literature is whether there is appetite and ability on the part of palliative care social workers to adopt and develop this role, and whether its culture enables or inhibits proactive steps forward. Many people refer to the classic phrase coined by the McKinsey organisation that culture is *how we do things around here* (Johnson *et al.*, 2013). While that may be true, there are so many elements that go into determining what you do and why. Whether you can define it or not, culture exists within organisations. It is the ethereal something that hangs in the air and influences how work gets done, it critically affects project success or failure and says who fits in and who does not. The research described in this paper attempts to redress this gap in the literature.

Methods

The context of the research was to consider the key challenges facing palliative care at a time of significant change, primarily from the perspective of its social workers. The focus of the research was on social work leadership at such a time within the palliative care sector and the degree to which the culture of palliative care social work may have had an impact on opportunities for social workers to serve as leaders.

The research took the form of a qualitative study undertaken from an Interpretivist perspective. It has been suggested that, social reality is something that is constructed and interpreted by people rather than something that exists objectively (Denscombe, 2002). Using this method

> can lead to significant advances in our theoretical understanding of social reality; more routinely, it is particularly good at enabling the researcher to learn, at first hand, about peoples perspectives on the subject chosen as the project focus (Davies, 2007).

The participants in the research were all deemed in my view to be 'leaders' in the field of end of life care. This judgement is based on the senior positions that they held within their organisations and/or within the sector. All bar one came from a social work background. For ethical reasons and to maintain anonymity the respondents were not named. All of the interviews were carried out in the respondent's place of work.

The selection process was straight forward. I identified individuals for interview, drawing on my own knowledge of the sector, or at the recommendation of others within my professional network.

The interview style that I chose of semi structured reflective interviews allowed for the use of open ended questions. Whilst this approach allowed the respondent to diverge from the interview topic it also offered the opportunity for new ways of seeing and understanding.

I focused on six questions in the course of the interview, designed to stimulate reflection and exploration. The questions were adapted from the work of Rank and Hutchinson (2000). Along with the work of Brilliant (1986), it was their theories that formed the foundations to the question for this research. The discussion of social work leadership began with Brilliant's (1986) analysis of social workers' resistance to take on leadership roles. She saw leadership as the missing ingredient in social work education but emphasised that leadership is an important aspect of the professional role for social workers. Analysing the roots of leadership as a non-theme in social work, she suggested that social work students were passionate about direct practice with clients, not with assuming leadership roles. Rank and Hutchinson (2000) carried out an analysis of leadership within the social work profession in the USA. They presented their results of a study which investigated how individuals in leadership positions perceived social work leadership.

The interview questions were specifically designed to test the leaders views against the theory base described in this literature.

Interview questions (adapted from Rank and Hutchinson, 2000):

(1) How do you define the concept of leadership within the context of end of life care?
(2) In your experience, do you perceive that social workers in end of life care embrace a concept of leadership?
(3) What do you believe are essential leadership skills and characteristics?
(4) What specific skills and qualities do you think social workers bring to the leadership table?
(5) Thinking generally, do you have any thoughts on how leadership could be promoted within palliative care social work?
(6) In your opinion, what pathway might a social worker have to take to become a leader in end of life care, like you?

All of the interviews were recorded electronically and transcribed verbatim. Their content was then analysed thematically. Thematic analysis is:

the study of the social meaning of tape recorded conversations – either naturally conducted or in an encounter with a research interviewer (Davies, 2007).

Identifying and classifying themes and then setting up a coding system was part of the analysis. The four main themes identified from the review of the literature were the historical, the political, and the cultural influences and leadership. I used a colour coding system, giving each theme a different colour and highlighted these in the transcription of each interview.

Throughout the course of the data collection and its analysis, I was aware that I was interacting with the research given my pre-exisiting role as a practicing social worker in end of life care. This epistemological stance may present some limitations to my objectivity of the data, but can be argued to be a strength in adding reflective depth and understanding to the data. It was important that I maintained a level of distance and continued to see the work from the eye of the researcher. This was particularly important to remember when carrying out the interviews and also when analysing the data. However, the very fact I was a practicing social worker meant I could take a reflective approach to the data and its analysis and interpretation.

The findings

Six leaders were selected and invited to be interviewed. All six agreed to take part. My assumption was that all of these leaders would have taken different paths to their own leadership and will have different ideas and interpretations as opposed to a single objective view. In other words my ontological assumption is that their reality would be subjective and vary between the participants.

The following chart lists the interviewees' positions and whether or not they were from a social work background.

Position held	Identifier	Social work background?
Senior manager in hospice care and national social care lead	Respondent A	Yes
Psychosocial lead in hospice care and senior academic	Respondent B	Yes
National social care lead for major UK charity	Respondent C	Yes
Hospice CEO	Respondent D	Yes
National end of life care lead for major UK charity	Respondent E	No
Senior academic in social work and chair of national eolc organisation.	Respondent F	Yes

There were four main influences identified from the literature review at the beginning of this research. These four influences then became a framework for the research and in particular the analysis and the interpretation of the findings. The influences were:

- *Historical* – Although in health and social care terms palliative care is a relatively modern day approach to care it has a long history spanning back to the late 1800s.
- *Political* – End of life care is higher on the health and social care agenda in the UK than it ever has been.
- *Cultural* – An interesting metaphor especially when applied to end of life care. When exploring the culture of hospices for example it could be suggested that the multi-disciplinary team (MDT) represents a series of sub cultures (i.e. nurses, doctors, social workers) working under a wider organisational culture.
- *Leadership* – 'Leadership is and must be socially critical, it does not reside in an individual but in the relationship between individuals, and it is oriented toward social vision and change, not simply, or only, organisational goals.' (Foster, 1989)

In my interpretation of the results, I have placed the influence of leadership at its centre, exploring the other influences from its perspective. The nature of leadership in palliative care is considered at the outset.

Leadership and palliative care social work

Respondents talked of the importance of leadership being exercised at all levels, however when talking about palliative care social workers respondent E said:

A lot of social workers do their evolution at a very low level. They do it at best by trying to influence MDT discussions but that will never make a leader of you. It might give you leadership in that context in that moment but in terms of really shaping the future of EOLC it needs to be done at both levels.

There was a real paradox in the data when respondents spoke of where social workers position themselves. In one way it was suggested that social workers are excluded, however it was also suggested that they exclude themselves and respondent C even went as far as to say:

There is a distinct tendency to play the oppressed minority card to themselves.

There was a suggestion that social workers choose to be less integrated:

social workers choose as teams very often not to be integrated into the organisations that they work in … one of the problems we have is that social work don't really want to be part of the hospice team but they also don't want to be part of the local authority so they sit in no mans land.

When talking about leadership, two of the respondents spoke about the need for leaders to be courageous and innovative and included in that the need for the leader to be comfortable with a certain level of disruptiveness.

It is about being courageous, thinking outside the box, it's about being innovative and … that's about being prepared to disrupt what's often very established processes and systems.

They also mentioned the need to take risks as well as the ability to assess risks. In fact one respondent went as far to say that:

'If you can take no risks then you cannot be a good leader'. They went onto say 'good leaders take quite high levels of risk but are knowledgeable about what the risks are and how they can be mitigated against if needed'. Another respondent said 'leadership is about taking people with you to do the difficult things'.

Most respondents talked about leaders in end of life care having to be honest, transparent and open. However one person said that although it was important to be honest it was also important for leaders to realise that there are some things you just do not share with the workforce or you have to choose the right time to disclose certain things. One respondent sums this up by saying *for me leadership has to come from the heart. It has to be visionary but it has to be meaningful.*

The respondents were asked to think about leadership specific to social workers working in end of life care. The data reveals that respondents found this a more difficult area to discuss. Not difficult in that they didn't have an opinion but difficult in that none of them could say that social workers necessarily embraced a concept of leadership. The data reveals this is not necessarily exclusive to palliative care social workers but a suggestion that social work as a profession overall may not embrace a concept of leadership. Different respondents gave different possible reasons for this.

Some interesting comments were made about how leadership is viewed within the social work profession. One respondent talked of credibility:

To be credible as a leader you have to understand what it's like to be a worker … leaders in social work are credible if they've worked up through the ranks, they've been there and done that. They understand the challenges.

Cultural influences

Out of the various influences considered it was 'culture' that seemed to dominate the discussions. There was more talk about the culture of palliative care social work than anything else.

Respondent D said:

there is a real psychological inhibition that lots of social workers have about asserting themselves as exercising any kind of leadership.

They go onto say:

it goes against the social work ethos of you're there to provide a service which should be around the patient and so they should be in charge not you … social work is about facilitating and enabling not about setting direction for other people.

The issue of power was mentioned when one of the respondents was talking about the social workers ability to take a systemic approach to leadership:

What social workers bring above all the other professions is a commitment to the systemic and that is really important. It's important in how you deal with service users in terms of understanding their context, who they are and where they've come from. It's important in terms of understanding other professions and how they come to the table. It's important in understanding the differences in power between groups and individuals, all of that they take a systemic approach.

However, another respondent said:

I think the focus on the individual becomes an excuse for never thinking at the systems level … that means then that social workers get to be the carping voice organisationally because they are seeking the best for their individual client and they choose not to think system, think organisation, think broader context, bring solutions to the table or bring options to the table.

There was some suggestion that due to the structure of hospices social workers are not considered as leaders. When talking about senior management teams in hospices respondent A said:

> The doctors can do it because they are in leadership positions from the word go. Within the definition of palliative care you must have a consultant so that's taken as red.

They go onto say:

> So what is that about? Is it like where you work with a taboo client group you become the taboo and if you work with a group of people who challenge the systems you are seen to be somebody that can't be worked on … its impossible for a social worker to do anything else because its not about a coat that you put on and take off.

Historical influences

> The past, present and future have important connections. It is necessary to explore the roots, foundations, fundamental policies and procedures relating to social work in palliative care (Harper, 2001).

Collating the historical findings revealed a real paradox in the responses of all respondents. When discussing EOLC and leadership all of the respondents answered in the present context but when talking about social work in EOLC almost all of the responses were stories and experiences of palliative care social work in the past.

Almost all respondents mentioned the work of Cicely Saunders and the impact she had on the modern hospice movement. Saunders was not only discussed within the context of leadership but also within the context of social work. One respondent said:

> Cicely Saunders conceived the idea of palliative care when she was a social worker but then had to become a doctor to make it happen.

When the respondents talked of the past history of the social work profession within the context of end of life care they described a very proactive group of individuals who were not only active within their services but were also active in research, writing academic papers and lobbying government with a view to shaping local and national policy.

Political influences

All six respondents mentioned the APCSW the national association set up in 1987 'representing the concerns and interests of both palliative care social workers and the patients and families with whom they work' (APCSW, 2013). However, there were expressions of confusion about the current role of the association. Respondent C talked about how *she never sees the association represented on the national stage and rarely hears its voice in answer to major issues facing the profession.*

When respondents spoke about the early days of the APCSW they used words like *radical, pioneers* and *courageous* to describe individual members. One said *In years gone by I think there were some amazing social workers who were pioneers.* However, when relating to modern day social workers most respondents talked about the sector having lost something.

In making reference to the wider social work profession currently in the UK respondent C said *where did the radical social workers go? Did they all get knackered in the 70s and just give up? What are we doing as professionals and as a profession?*

Conversely, many of the respondents also spoke of a proud tradition in palliative care social work. Almost all respondents used the example of how in the past these radical, courageous pioneers lobbied national government and were successful in changing welfare benefit policy with the introduction of the DS1500 (a special rules criteria for those with a prognosis of 6 months or less to be fast tracked for high rate Personal Independent Payment), something which is still in use today. Respondent E said:

> I think collectively there is quite a proud tradition in palliative care social work. I think there is a tradition of campaigning. I think it is probably the one area of social work where there is a tradition of teaching and leading by communicating the ethos of palliative care.

Another issue which almost all respondents talked about was the challenge in palliative care social work of being able to evidence its worth and merit in the delivery of end of life care. This has been an issue for the profession for a long time but respondents spoke of it being particularly relevant in the current climate of commissioning services. Respondent C said:

> There isn't evidence as to what palliative care social work does, so without that evidence we can't extol the virtues of it. At the moment it's a self dooming prophecy that it's a dying profession and yes it is because we can't prove our worth.

There were several quotes on the current position of EOLC in the wider health and social care landscape which revealed a need for a social work voice. Some examples of these are:

> Never before has there been such a key role for the influence of social care

> Why social workers shouldn't see themselves as the central role in thinking about how to work with patients and develop services is something of a mystery

> The more we get into this notion of developing communities and supporting an increased use of volunteering the more that brings palliative care closer towards our core professional framework than ever

> I think the future of EOLC is about a social model but unless we have some social workers that are strong leaders it won't get a chance

Discussion

For the purposes of this paper, this discussion focuses on the questions of whether social workers in palliative care should aspire to a position of leadership and if so how they achieve this. Given the heavy focus on cultural influences on the question of social workers as leaders, this is given particular attention in this section of the paper.

Social workers should aspire to be leaders in palliative care

There is strong evidence from the research that leadership in palliative care on the part of social workers involved in the sector is an aspiration to be pursued.

One of the respondents in this research made reference to palliative care social work in the United States having recently been out to a palliative care social work conference in the US where leadership was high on their agenda. She said:

> there were 250 people all of whom are incredibly well qualified, doing some really innovative and coherent pieces of work ... there was a level of enthusiasm ... a community and a get up and go in the room that I think we haven't got at the moment.

Background to this research confirms significant changes in how terminal illness and bereavement are viewed and experienced. They are social issues rather than a series of medical problems, they are events that are highly individual in nature, and they are often particularly complex for people who are marginalised. What better context for the social work perspective at related strategic discussions? Add in a political agenda around integration between health and social care services and the argument is further strengthened. Social workers would bring a unique, and much needed voice about how these issues are best addressed as services are developed and refined. This was the view of many of the respondents I interviewed who talked about such gaps in care provision and related strategy. They were clear that in their view these gaps would be best addressed by the voice and considerations of social work leaders given the values and priorities held by the profession. Their views would be best heard and acted upon if social workers were in positions of leadership.

By the same token, they also warned that if these gaps are not filled by social work leaders then they *just get filled by others*. The gaps were also referred to as 'the space' and it was suggested that *social workers might even be frightened or reticent to claim the space*.

Many of the respondents made reference to the values held by social workers as an important reason for requiring that social workers are involved in strategic decisions.

However, it is exactly these values that could be preventing social workers from embracing a concept of leadership.

> Professions such as nursing and teaching have identified a crisis of leadership and have instigated successful strategic initiatives and programs to develop leaders and leadership. However, social work has been less proactive and even reluctant in taking on leadership as an issue for theory and practice (McDonald, 2009).

McDonald goes on to say:

> in our view social work has actually recoiled from the idea of leadership, harbouring an historical view that leadership is somehow contradictory to social work values and its underlying philosophy.

The interview findings reveal stark contrast between descriptions of the radical social workers of the past and the less courageous social workers of today. There is a suggestion that social workers working in the specialty currently are focused on doing things according to policy and by regulation and work in a bounded way. This is somewhat at odds with literature describing leadership, which confirms that leaders must be willing to cross boundaries and push against them. The radical social workers of the past, who did indeed pushed boundaries and drove changes in policy and regulation, appear to embody that particular aspect of being a leader. It appears an approach to change that is at odds with social work practice today.

Clarity about the strategic role and future agenda of social workers in palliative care would be helpful

Lack of clarity about the role may be linked to the apparent absence of a strong strategic agenda to which palliative care social workers might be working. If they do not perceive leadership within their role then they are unlikely to feel it their responsibility to set an agenda, even one that draws heavily on their skills, for the sector. One respondent spoke about the potential consequences for some very promising developments if social workers are not in a position to rise to the challenge.

> I think the future of end of life care is about a social model but unless we have some social workers that are strong leaders it won't get a chance.

If the future of end of life care is about a social model then arguably it is up to the profession to establish a related agenda to focus future thinking, partnerships and collaborations. However, there is currently no evidence to suggest that such thoughts and preparations are underway. In contrast, the evidence from this study and my experience does suggest a lack of leadership and strategic thinking. With stronger leadership within the profession senior practitioners along with their teams could develop, at a strategic level, a professional agenda fit for the future. Participants in my study confirmed a belief in even greater impact if a group of leaders from social work could be persuaded to work together and act on behalf of the profession of palliative care social work as a whole.

Senior social workers in palliative care need to be more engaged in debate

Decisions about the future shape, funding and delivery of palliative care are far from straightforward. They are being deliberated in a variety of fora, to inform policy and practice. They would benefit from multiple perspectives and careful thought.

Participants in this research confirmed the opportunity that this presented to social work, and indeed a need for this group to be present in such discussions. However, they described how in their experience there was often a vacuum, a space, a missing link in their discussions about the future of end of life care in the UK, specifically a strong voice representing social care. In their experience social care is often reluctant to put its head above the parapet and engage in these conversations.

As a result, this space is filled by other professions, so then when new thinking and new work streams are made public, options that would incorporate the unique offering of palliative care social workers have not been developed.

Social workers interested in leadership need training and opportunities to build their careers

It is clear that whilst some leadership is exercised by social work on a number of levels, and particularly in relation to operational issues there is a lack of formal leadership development for palliative care social workers.

Brilliant (1986) revealed similar gaps in social work education over twenty years ago and as the literature reveals not much has changed since then. How can we expect palliative care social workers to step into leadership roles without the relevant support, experience, training and education? Education or other development opportunities will not be sufficient or indeed appropriately shaped without greater clarity and definition of the role that social workers should fulfill in the future. Whether lack of education and other development opportunities is a result of, or contributes to the lack of career progression is unclear. However, all participants in this research talked about how limited opportunities were for social workers to progress in their careers.

This, linked with the cultural and historical findings, suggests that social workers are not considered as leaders in the sector. The interview findings also revealed a flat structure in palliative care social work that does not lend itself to people climbing the ranks and progressing through their careers.

Greater evidence about the unique contribution of the palliative care social worker would support their role as a leader

A significant challenge highlighted by almost all respondents focused on the requirement being made of all professionals including palliative care social workers to provide evidence of their worth and merit in the EOLC sector today. This is not a new ask of the profession but respondents spoke of it as being particularly relevant in the current climate, giving the growing interest of commissioners in outcomes. Paradoxically this is arguably very difficult to achieve without strong leaders within the profession and the sector. New work on outcome measures is being undertaken by a number of institutions (for example the OACC initiative run by the Cicely Saunders Institute, London), but the question regarding the degree to which such measures capture data pertinent to the social workers role has enjoyed little public debate. If its outcome measures are deemed to be valuable in confirming improvements on the part of patients or carers attributable to social workers, then the profession should be pushing for their greater use.

Social workers need to influence the culture in which they work

There is some evidence that the culture of palliative care social work is changing. In 2015 the APCSW at their annual conference launched potential designs for their new logo and website in partnership with a leading business design consultancy firm. They also announced that their executive committee was working on a strategy for palliative care social work which would be ready for consultation in 2016. This is an ideal opportunity for the association to support the profession to see leadership as empowerment, as enablement, as a way of ensuring that all the things that guide palliative care social workers in their practice with patients and families can be perpetuated, amplified, developed and embedded in whole models of care.

Achieving this requires strong leadership by social care professionals. This research suggests social workers can and do influence at all levels. Social workers need to use this leadership behaviour to positively influence organisational outcomes, think of ways to create pathways to leadership and become role models for both their own profession and the wider multi professional teams in which they work.

Conclusion

This research confirms that the profession of palliative care social work is seen to have a vital role in the development and provision of end of life care services and that its members have a very strong and proud tradition on which to build. However it also suggests that palliative care social work does not have a strong enough presence at a strategic level and because of this puts itself at risk. In turn this puts the care and support required by growing numbers of people who are dying in the UK at risk.

If the profession of palliative care social work as a whole does not take responsibility for this then they risk that gap being filled by another professional group and their voice becoming silent.

Strong social work leadership is an important missing ingredient in the current mix. If it were to be added to the growing efforts of many to improve end of life care at local, regional and national levels its potential impact could be increased further. It is time for palliative care social workers to engage in strategies individually and collectively that will enable them to take their rightful place along with other professionals at discussions where strategic direction, relationships and action are being considered. It is no longer time to talk about what is being missed but to demonstrate its added value. There is an empty chair at that table. It's time for palliative care social workers to take that seat.

Disclosure statement

No potential conflict of interest was reported by the authors.

References

Brilliant, E. L. (1986) 'Social work leadership: a missing ingredient?', *Social Work*, vol. 31, pp. 325–331.

Davies, M. (2007) *Doing a successful research project: Using qualitative or quantitative methods*, Palgrave Macmillan, Basingstoke.

Denscombe, M. (2007) *Groundrules for good research: A 10 point guide for social researchers*, Open University Press, Buckingham.

Hospice UK. (2012) Commission into the Future of Hospice Care. *Preparing for the Future: Key Operating Principles*. Hospice UK, London.

Independent Review of the Liverpool Care Pathway. (2013) *More care, less pathway*, A review of the Liverpool Care Pathway, Independent Review of the Liverpool Care Pathway, London.

Johnson, G., Whittington, R., Scholes, K., Angwin, D. & Regnér, P. (2013). *Exploring Strategy: Text and Cases*. (10th ed) Pearson, Harlow.

Leadbeater, C. & Garber, J. (2010) *Dying for Change*, DEMOS, London.

National End of Life Care Programme. (2010) *Supporting People to Live and Die Well: A Framework for Social Care at the End of Life*.

Rank, M. G. & Hutchinson, W. S. (2000) 'An analysis of leadership within the social work profession', *Journal of Social Work Education*, vol. 36, no. 3, pp. 487–502.

Schein, E. (2010) *Organisational Culture and Leadership*, Jossey-Bass, Wiley, San Francisco, CA.

Anne Cullen

SCHWARTZ ROUNDS® – PROMOTING COMPASSIONATE CARE AND HEALTHY ORGANISATIONS

This article reviews evidence about the factors that can make it difficult for healthcare staff to provide compassionate care for individuals and their families. These relate to the intrinsic strain of caring for people who are suffering both physically and existentially, and the pressure of working conditions including high workloads, lack of support and continuing change. It presents Schwartz Rounds as an intervention that responds directly to these factors and has been found to be of significant benefit in hospitals, hospices and other health care settings in the USA and UK. It describes how this intervention is based on techniques that are integral to the practice of many social workers and draws attention to the fact that palliative care social workers have played a significant role in establishing the rounds in end of life services. It suggests that Schwartz Rounds could be helpfully introduced in other areas of activity where social workers and others are employed to provide care and protection for vulnerable people, including children and young people, where similar pressures and limitations have been identified.

1. Introduction

'The tension between the intended moral and ethical purpose of care and the inevitable day-to-day difficulties of retaining that purpose at the point of care is a shared dilemma of all in health care …' (Goodrich and Cornwell, 2008, p. 3).

This quotation highlights the difficulties that all of us face as practitioners and managers in health and social care in holding on not only to the ideals and aspirations that brought us into this work but also to the crucial ability to connect with the people that we care for at the level of a fellow human being, to see 'the person in the patient' (Goodrich and Cornwell, 2008). The consequences of losing this ability have been forcefully highlighted in relation to end of life care by the recent report by the Parliamentary and Health Service Ombudsman (2015), which draws attention to a series of examples of cases where dying people and their families have been failed by both primary care and hospital services.

This article reviews evidence about the factors that can impair the ability of staff to provide compassionate care for individuals and their families with a particular focus on end of life care.

It presents Schwartz Rounds® (sometimes referred to as Schwartz Center Rounds®) as an intervention that responds directly to these factors and has been found to be of significant benefit in hospitals, hospices and other health care settings in the USA and UK. It notes that this intervention is based on techniques that are integral to the practice of many social workers and that in practice palliative care social workers have played a significant role in establishing the rounds in end of life services. It suggests that Schwartz Rounds® could be helpfully introduced in other areas of activity where social workers and others are employed to provide care and protection for vulnerable people, including children and young people.

2. The problem of sustaining compassionate care

In a recent report commissioned by Hospice UK Goodrich *et al.* (2015) identify two overarching sources of stress that are experienced by people working in health services: Firstly, the intrinsic nature of the work or 'emotional labour' of caring for people who are suffering, physically and existentially. In the context of end of life services Goodrich *et al.* observe that that: 'Continuous contact with patients who are ill, in distress and dying means that staff … are constantly confronting their own mortality and vulnerability.' They note that the term 'compassion', which is derived from Latin, means literally 'suffering with', which highlights that being compassionate is by its very nature emotionally demanding (p. 15).

The second cause of health worker stress that the authors identify is their working conditions. They observe that in NHS hospital trusts particularly there is a strong emphasis on targets and financial efficiency and an imperative to move patients through services quickly. This means that staffs who are working in large, busy, pressured environments have less opportunity than previously to establish relationships with either patients or colleagues. Combined with high workloads, demanding time pressures, limited support and low levels of involvement in decision-making this can place individuals at risk of becoming 'burnt out' or in other words demotivated and emotionally detached from the people they care for.

It might reasonably be expected that people working in hospices would experience especially high levels of stress because they are continually in the presence of death and loss. Goodrich *et al.* report, however, that hospice staff are no more stressed than those in other care settings, possibly because despite these pressures there are also some particularly rewarding features of the work. From the author's own experience these include the satisfactions of working in a setting where standards of practice are consistently high and the appreciation that is expressed by many patients and relatives. Despite this Goodrich *et al.* comment that people who work in hospices are still vulnerable to stress because in spite of such rewards they are repeatedly witnessing or 'suffering with' people in distress. Additionally, and in common with people in many other care settings, hospice staff are often working hard but invisibly to present a calm and hopeful exterior in order to protect patients, relatives and colleagues from the burden of their own distress and uncertainty.

Goodrich *et al.* go on to draw attention to reports, such as those produced by Help the Hospices (2013), which highlight anticipated changes in demography that are likely to increase the pressures experienced not only by hospice staff but by all health and social care staff working with people coming to the end of their lives. As people live longer and develop multiple health problems that may affect both their physical and mental health simultaneously, the demands for sophisticated and extended end of life care will grow. This coincides with, and indeed exacerbates a situation in which both personal and public funds are increasingly squeezed. It creates an imperative for organisations across the spectrum of health and social care to make radical changes to the way in which services are organised and delivered: to provide more care at home, to make more use of technology and to increase the involvement of volunteers and family carers in providing forms of care that would previously have been undertaken by paid staff. Importantly, they note that making significant changes in the way that people work is in itself known to be a significant source of stress.

More positively, however, Goodrich *et al.* draw attention to evidence that taking positive steps to support staff can enhance their resilience and with it their ability to sustain quality of care even under pressure. Particularly powerful evidence comes from a recent large scale, three year mixed method research project for the National Institute for Health Research (Maben *et al.*, 2012) which explored the experience of NHS patients and staff in both hospital and community settings. This showed that where organisations took proactive measures to support staff this not only improved their wellbeing but was associated with better quality of patient care. One of the key messages from this study was that 'Seeking systematically to enhance staff wellbeing is not only important in its own right but also for the quality of patient experiences' (Maben *et al.*, 2012, p. 4).

In the next section of this article I will describe Schwartz Rounds® and in the following one I will present evidence that they can be an effective means of providing staff support that is responsive to both the intrinsic stress of caring for dying people and the challenges posed by working conditions.

3. Schwartz Rounds®

Schwartz Rounds® are named in honour of Kenneth Schwartz, a medical lawyer who was based in Boston, USA. In 1994 at the age of 40 he was diagnosed with advanced adenocarcinoma of the lung. In an article written only weeks before he died in 1995 he described how in the months following his diagnosis, 'I was subjected to chemotherapy, radiation therapy, surgery, and news of all kinds, most of it bad', but that crucially 'the ordeal has been punctuated by moments of exquisite compassion', in the form of 'acts of kindness — the simple human touch from my caregivers', which, 'have made the unbearable bearable' (Schwartz, 1995).

Schwartz's legacy became the Schwartz Center for Compassionate Healthcare[1], which introduced Schwartz Rounds® in 1997 as a means by which, 'Caregivers have an opportunity to share their experiences, thoughts and feelings on thought-provoking topics drawn out from actual patient cases.' The reason why this is felt to be important is 'the premise … that caregivers are better able to make personal connections with patients and colleagues when they have greater insight into their own responses and feelings,' (Schwartz Center for Compassionate Care website, quoted in Mullick *et al.*, 2013).

Rounds now run in 375 healthcare sites across the USA.[2] In 2009 they were introduced in the UK by the Point of Care Programme (now the Point of Care Foundation) in two hospital pilot sites. Following a positive evaluation Schwartz Rounds® have been rolled out across over 100 healthcare settings, including 26 hospices.[3]

The following description of what happens in a Schwartz round draws on the handbook provided for sites introducing Schwartz Rounds® (Point of Care Foundation, 2013), my own experience as a Schwartz Round facilitator and mentor to new sites and ideas generated within mentor workshops provided by the Point of Care Foundation. Within the description I include commentary to try to show how rounds incorporate concepts and methods from therapeutic practice that will be familiar to many social workers.

Schwartz Rounds® are based on the model of a hospital Grand Round, where a clinical team presents a case and treatment plan for discussion with clinical peers from other departments. A major difference, however, is that the focus of Schwartz Rounds® is on the personal experience of staff in the course of carrying out their jobs: the psychological and emotional impact on them as human beings. Schwartz Rounds® are emphatically not forums for solving practical problems but rather protected spaces for reflection. A further important difference is that Rounds® are open to all staff, not only doctors, nurses, allied health professionals, psychosocial and spiritual care practitioners but also cleaners, porters, maintenance workers, office staff, managers, board members and volunteers.

Food is provided beforehand as a practical demonstration of the nurturing function of the round. Rounds are co-facilitated by a psychosocial facilitator and a medical lead. The former may be a clinical psychologist, social worker, psychotherapist or sometimes a nurse or other clinician with relevant specialist skills. In hospices this role is often undertaken by a specialist palliative care social worker, as it is in a small number of hospitals. The medical lead is usually a senior doctor.

At the start of the round the psychosocial facilitator sets the 'ground rules' for the round. This action and the content of the rules themselves amounts to a process of creating the 'frame' for the session that has much in common with the conditions of a therapy or clinical supervision session (Langs, 1982; Jordan and Marshall, 2010). Its function is to set up the round as a relatively safe, consistent and predictable environment or, in therapeutic terms 'a space in which unbearable feelings and unthinkable thoughts can be safely confronted and explored (Ruch, 2010, p.43).

The facilitator explains that the round is confidential, that it will last for precisely one hour and that its purpose is to share and reflect on the personal and emotional impact of the work. She/he advises participants that they will be expected to refrain from trying to come up with practical solutions, tempting as that may be. She/he then sets out the format for the round: A panel of presenters (usually two to four people) will speak for 15–20 min in total; after which the round will be opened for discussion. Towards the end of that time the facilitator will come back to the panel to invite them, if they wish, to respond to what has been said during the round and add any final thoughts.

Throughout the round the facilitators continue to hold the frame. This includes managing the time and gently steering participants away from probing presenters for clinical details that are not relevant to the focus of the round or attempting to come up with practical solutions.

A second therapy derived feature is the stance that the facilitators model in their own behaviour and encourage others to adopt throughout the round. Although this is sometimes referred to in the Schwartz literature as a 'neutral' one it is more accurately the position that Cecchin has characterised as that of 'respectful curiosity' (Cecchin, 1987). This is significant because it highlights an important source of the energy, insight and creativity that can be generated within Rounds®.

The stance of respectful curiosity comes from within the systemic school of family therapy (Walsh, 2011). This adopts a post-modernist, social constructionist perspective, which suggests that the social world of any group or organisation, i.e. what people say and do and feel, is not only the product of formal structures, rules and procedures but also of the way that people talk about and make sense of their experiences, to themselves and one another. The stance of respectful curiosity is used to encourage different members of, for example, a family, team or organisation to give their account of an experience or relationship from their own unique perspective, and to promote a process of listening, exploring, extending and deepening the accounts and making connections between them. This can open up possibilities for productive change in how people feel and act in relation to both themselves and other people. This in turn can help to bring about significant changes in how effectively the family, team or organisation functions, including how well it promotes the wellbeing of its members. It is important to the process that each account is listened to with similar respect, irrespective of the relative status of the individual concerned, because each of these personal narratives adds detail and texture to the understanding of what is going on and to the resource of ideas available to stimulate change (Carr, 2006).

What happens in a Schwartz Round is a similar process: people are invited and supported to tell and explore their stories about their own experiences, to listen, be curious about and reflect on those of others and to make connections between them.

This process begins after the facilitator's introduction, when the presenters are invited to give their own perspective on a particular case or theme, focusing on how it has impacted on them from a personal and emotional point of view. Presenters speak informally without visual aids. Rounds often focus on an experience where a clinical team or group of staff were faced with a patient or family situation that was particularly challenging or disturbing. Titles of such rounds might be on the lines of 'Caught between the patient and the family' or 'Dying too young'. Other rounds may be theme based, for example, 'A colleague/patient I'll never forget', 'Why am I here?', 'My worst day at work'.

Following the presentation the facilitators hand the discussion over to the people who up till then have been the audience for the presentations, inviting them to ask exploratory questions of the panel, to voice what they have been feeling as they listened to the presentations or to talk about experiences of their own that may have been brought to mind by what they have heard.

Throughout the session the facilitators work to deepen the discussion and to help participants to surface meaning. They may, for example, gently probe a speaker whose contribution seems to carry a high level of emotional charge to try to elicit the experience that lies behind it. They may articulate themes that they detect beneath the surface of the discussion. In keeping with the systemic, social constructionist perspective these are offered provisionally, as possibilities that participants may choose to take up or to leave as they choose (Carr, 2006).

At the end of the round facilitators thank the presenters and the audience for their contributions and offer a brief personal commentary on what has taken place within the round. Again this is offered not as an authoritative summation but as a particular take on what has gone on that people may wish to take away and reflect on or not as they prefer.

One brief example from my own experience as a hospice Schwartz Round facilitator illustrates the two therapeutic dynamics that I have attempted to describe: firstly, providing containment to explore 'unbearable feelings' and 'unthinkable thoughts'; secondly, eliciting and making productive connections between different personal and professional stories of people within the organisation.

A round was entitled, 'There's nothing you can do to help'. It focused on experiences of working with people in the late stages of Motor Neurone Disease (MND). Three presenters spoke about how they each felt that they had failed these people even though in each case it was evident that the relevant circumstances were beyond their own control. The presenters in the room were themselves surprised at the number of other colleagues who told their own stories and it became clear that there were multiple variations on this theme of how defeated people often felt in relation to this particularly cruel disease. There was some sense of relief within the round that people had been able to talk about their personal distress and sense of professional inadequacy but also a deep sadness.

After the round another narrative emerged, however. Through a member of the steering group that organises the rounds it was fed back that someone from an area of work outside the clinical service had attended the round, without realising what the topic of the round was going to be. This person had a close relative who was suffering from MND. They had been inevitably upset by what they had heard but reported that they had taken great comfort from the evidence that even when their clinical colleagues felt helpless they continued to care and do their best for these individuals and their families.

4. Impact

Round attendees are routinely requested to complete evaluation forms, contributing to a substantial body of data about the impact of Rounds® within different types of organisations. Attendance at hospital Schwartz Rounds® in the UK can be over 100 (Wren, 2014). Hospices are much smaller organisations so numbers are lower in total, although not proportionally. Reed et al. (2014) for example report mean average attendance at the first 12 Rounds® in a hospice of 44 (range 31–57). Both hospital and hospice sites Rounds® are consistently highly rated, e.g. Reed et al. report that 78% of respondents rated Rounds® as excellent or exceptional and that 87% of respondents reported that they had gained insight into how others think and feel in relation to caring for patients.

There have been a number of evaluation studies and a multi-site, multi-element independent study is currently in progress in the UK under the auspices of National Institute for Health Research.[4] This section draws on five published sources to seek to provide a summary of the evidence to date of the impact of Schwartz Rounds®. These sources are: an independent evaluation of Schwartz Rounds® in the USA conducted by Lown and Manning (2010); the Point of Care evaluation of the two hospital pilots of Schwartz Rounds® in the UK (Goodrich, 2012); a report on the experience of introducing rounds in a UK hospice (Mullick et al., 2013); findings from a small multi-method evaluation of Schwartz Rounds® in another UK hospice (Reed et al., 2014); and a reflective paper by Wren (2014), again written on the basis of experience of Schwartz Rounds® in the UK.

4.1. Support and validation

Goodrich describes how senior staff saw Schwartz Rounds® as a mechanism through which they could demonstrate a corporate understanding of the connection between the core purpose of the service and the importance of staff care, 'we are here to care for patients so we need to look after staff' (Goodrich, 2012, p. 121). Reciprocally, all of the sources report that in practice staff who attended rounds felt more supported by their organisation, simply by being provided with this forum and the message of concern for their welfare that it conveyed.

The reports show that participants valued the opportunity that rounds provided to speak openly about their own painful experiences and feelings, but that in addition finding resonances of these in the accounts of presenters and other participants served to validate their experiences and reduce their sense of isolation. Lown and Manning, Goodrich and Wren all note that other staff were particularly impressed and touched when senior managers and doctors who normally presented as being confident and authoritative were willing to talk about situations where they felt that they had made mistakes or failed people. Wren comments that hearing such accounts could help people to feel more compassionate towards themselves and their own perceived limitations.

Lown and Manning's USA study, which evaluated sites where rounds had been running for much longer than in the UK sites, found evidence that attending rounds had improved participants' ability to provide responsive care. One of their key findings was that respondents reported that they were able to be more empathetic to the needs of the people they cared for because they had become more emotionally aware and gained insight into the psychological and social aspects of their patients' lives. This meant that they were better able to pick up cues from patients and follow these up by asking questions that helped them to identify and meet patients' needs better. They also reported that they were more aware of the presence of family members and more active in offering them support. With this enhanced interest and confidence in engaging with the 'person in the patient' came renewed energy and enthusiasm for the work. Particularly encouragingly Lown and Manning found consistent evidence that these benefits increased with the number of rounds that the contributors to the evaluation had attended.

4.2. Sense of connection

All of the sources report that participants gained from hearing people from other roles and sections of the organisation talking about their work. This included, for example, an enhanced appreciation of the burden of responsibility carried by medical staff (Lown and Manning, 2010) and a more vivid and detailed picture of the work undertaken by people in non-clinical roles (Mullick et al., 2013; Reed et al., 2014).

An important associated gain reported was that rounds gave people a new and more rewarding perspective in being able to locate themselves as part of a collective enterprise. 'The mosaic … is more clear, instead of … being in your own encapsulated environment (Lown and Manning, 2010, p. 1078). 'I sometimes feel as if you're a little part of a jigsaw and going to a Schwartz Round you see all the other bits of the jigsaw, so you actually get the whole picture … it's reassuring, … it's educational … it's enlightening' (Reed *et al.*, 2014, p. 2).

These enhanced insights helped people to feel more connected to individual colleagues, the overall purpose of the organisation and,as Wren expresses it, 'the values that motivated them to enter healthcare' (Wren, 2014, p. 23).

4.3.   Practical changes

As well as enhanced confidence in approaching and interacting with colleagues from other teams informally, Lown and Manning's evaluation identifies that over time what people have heard within rounds can lead conversations outside them that result in productive changes in both working practices and service delivery structures. Examples include more timely referrals to palliative care services on one site and a restructuring from single profession to multi-disciplinary teams on anther, because what doctors had heard in rounds had educated them about the specific skills that could be provided by colleagues from other professions.

4.4.   A realistic organisational narrative

Wren makes the further important observation that over time Rounds® can help people across an organisation to develop more realistic expectations and accommodate to unavoidable limitations. She notes that many rounds are about situations in which health care professionals were unable to 'make it better' or how the organisation has failed to protect staff from something that has damaged them. She observes that:

Rounds discussions often contain an underlying hope that there is a policy or strategy that will deal with this and that the organisations 'must' be able to protect them. Over time the Rounds help the community of staff to digest the fact that there isn't, it can't and to reflect on and appreciate how they are withstanding painful situations — and surviving in cases where it would be difficult to thrive (Wren, 2014, p. 24).

5.   Conclusion

The material presented in the last section highlights the various ways in which Schwartz Rounds® can contribute to sustaining the resilience that people working in end of life services need in order to be able to provide compassionate and responsive care under what are likely to be increasingly challenging conditions. They show that rounds can provide staff with support and validation of painful experiences; an enhanced appreciation and sense of connection with colleagues, and with the purpose of the service as a whole; and the opportunity to have a voice in conversations that can change working practices and improve care. Additionally, they can provide a means for people to come together from across the different roles and hierarchies within the organisation to develop a realistic and coherent, continually evolving narrative about the possibilities and the limitations of the care and support they can provide for the people they serve and for each other.

At the end of the article I would like suggest that Schwartz Rounds® might helpfully be adopted in other areas of service where social workers and colleagues from other disciplines are employed to provide care and protection for other vulnerable people, including children and young people. There are striking parallels between the sources of stress that Goodrich, Harrison and Cornwell identify in relation in hospital trusts and those identified by the final report of the Munro Review of Child Protection Services (2011). As Lees, Meyer and Rafferty observe (2011) this report describes how social workers' anxiety and distress at being repeatedly exposed to 'suffering, deprivation and need' (p. 14) is compounded by working conditions in which they experience high levels of bombardment and low levels of control, with serious consequences for their ability to achieve adequate and reliable standards of professional practice.

At a time when the prospects for the future of social work and social care are at least as challenging and uncertain as they are in health services Schwartz Rounds® appear to represent a relatively economical and worthwhile source of support. The recent resurgence of interest in the relational and therapeutic aspects of the social work role (Ruch, 2010), the move to 'Reclaim' social work (Goodman and Trowler, 2011), and the introduction of principal social workers in all local authorities to champion excellence in social work practice mean that there should be a growing number of social workers who are equipped with the skills to follow the lead provided by palliative care social workers in introducing rounds into their organisations and acting as facilitators for them.

Disclosure statement

No potential conflict of interest was reported by the author.

Notes

1. http://www.theschwartzcenter.org.
2. Schwartz Center for Compassionate Healthcare http://www.theschwartzcenter.org/supporting-caregivers/schwartz-center-rounds. Accessed 26 May 2015.
3. Information from Point of Care Foundation http://www.pointofcarefoundation.org.uk/schwartz-rounds Accessed 26.5.2015.
4. http://www.nets.nihr.ac.uk/projects/hsdr/130,749.

References

Carr, A. (2006) 'The consultation process and intake interviews', in *The Handbook of Child and Adolescent Psychology: A Contextual Approach*, Routledge, London.

Cecchin, G. (1987) 'Hypothesizing, circularity, and neutrality revisited: an invitation to curiosity', *Family Process*, vol. 26, no. 4, pp. 405–413.

Goodman, S. & Trowler, I. (2011) *Social Work Reclaimed*, Jessica Kingsley, London.

Goodrich, J. & Cornwell, J. (2008) *Seeing the Person in the Patient*, King's Fund, London.

Goodrich, J. (2012) 'Supporting hospital staff to provide compassionate care: Do Schwartz Center Rounds work in English hospitals?', *Journal of the Royal Society of Medicine*, vol. 105, pp. 117–122.

Goodrich, J., Harrison, T. & Cornwell, C. (2015) *Resilience: A Framework for Hospice Staff to Flourish in Stressful Times*, Hospice UK, London.

Help the Hospices Commission. (2013) *Future Needs and Preferences for Hospice Care: Challenges and Opportunities for Hospices*, Help the Hospices, London.

Jordan, M. & Marshall, H. (2010) 'Taking counselling and psychotherapy outside: destruction of the therapeutic frame?', *European Journal of Psychotherapy & Counselling*, vol. 14, no. 4, pp. 345–359.

Langs, R. (1982) *Psychotherapy: A Basic Text*, Jason Aronson, Northvale, NJ.

Lees, A., Meyer, E., Rafferty, J. (2013) 'From Menzies Lyth to Munro: the problem of managerialism', *British Journal of Social Work*, vol. 42, no. 3, pp. 542–558.

Lown, B. & Manning, C. (2010) 'The Schwartz Center Rounds: evaluation of an interdisciplinary approach to enhancing patient-centred communication', *Teamwork and Provider Support, Academic Medicine*, vol. 85, no. 6, pp. 1073–1081.

Maben, J., Peccei, R., Adams, M., Robert, G., Richardson, A., Murrells, T. & Morrow, E. (2012) *Patients' Experiences of Care and the Influence of Staff Motivation, Affect and Wellbeing. Final Report*, NIHR Service Delivery and Organisation programme, Southampton.

Mullick, A., Wright, A., Watmore-Eve, J. & Flatley, M. (2013) 'Supporting hospice staff: the introduction of Schwartz Center Rounds® to a UK hospice setting', *European Journal of Palliative Care*, vol. 20, no. 2, pp. 62–65.

Parliamentary and Health Service Ombudsman. (2015) *Dying without Dignity*. Available from: http://www.ombudsman.org.uk/reports-and-consultations/reports/health/dying-without-dignity [Accessed 25 May 2015].

Munro, E., (2011) *The Munro Review of Child Protection: Final Report*, Department for Education, London.

Point of Care Foundation. (2013) *Setting up and Running Schwartz Center Rounds®*, Point of Care Foundation, London.

Reed, E., Cullen, A., Gannon, C., Knight, A. & Todd, J. (2014) 'Use of Schwartz Centre Rounds in a UK hospice: findings from a longitudinal evaluation', *Journal of Interprofessional Care*, vol. 25, pp. 1–2.

Ruch, G.. (2010) 'Theoretical frameworks informing relationship based practice', in *Relationship Based Social Work: Getting to the Heart of Practice*, eds G. Ruch, D. Turney & A. Ward, Jessica Kingsley, London.

Schwartz, K.B. (1995). A patient's story, *Boston Globe Magazine*, Jul 16. Available from: http://www.theschwartzcenter.org/about-us/story-mission [Accessed 26 May 2015].

Walsh, F. (2011) 'Theory and practice in clinical social work', in *Theory and Practice in Clinical Social Work*, ed J. Brandell, Sage, Los Angeles, CA.

Wren, B. (2014) 'Schwartz rounds: "an intervention with potential to simultaneously improve staff experience and organisational culture"', *Clinical Psychology Forum*, vol. 263, pp. 22–25.

Index